Contents

CHILD OBESITY

A Parent's Guide

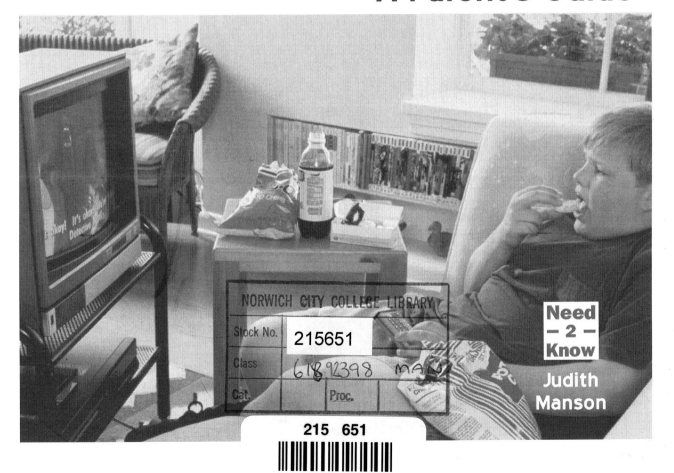

Need
— 2 —
Know

Judith
Manson

First published in Great Britain in 2008 by
Need2Know
Remus House
Coltsfoot Drive
Peterborough
PE2 9JX
Telephone 01733 898103
Fax 01733 313524
www.n2kbooks.com

Need2Know is an imprint of Forward Press Ltd.
www.forwardpress.co.uk
SB ISBN 978-1-86144-049-5
Cover photograph: Donna Day, Stone, Getty Images

Introduction

Experts agree that the 'obesity time bomb' is currently the most serious threat to our children's health and it's not going to go away. But with the right help, advice and support, everyone can help children eat well, keep active and live a happy and healthy life.

This book is for parents, grandparents, guardians and carers of children ranging from toddlers to teenagers. It will also be of interest to teachers, professional childcare workers or anyone who is concerned about children's health and the current hot topic of child obesity. It sets out clearly and simply, the facts about obesity and what you can do to help children tackle it.

Obesity rates in the UK have been rising at an alarming rate; obesity in children has more than trebled in the past twenty years with 10 per cent of six-year-olds and 17 per cent of all teenagers now classified as obese. If the trend continues, by 2020 half of all British children will be obese.

This topic is rarely out of the news these days and you could say there is almost a media epidemic about the obesity epidemic. Much of the information is alarming and lots of parents are becoming worried about their children and want to know the facts behind the headlines and statistics. Also younger and younger children are now picking up on body image and becoming confused a lot earlier in their lives about what represents a healthy size and weight.

Because obesity is so high profile in the media, there's a greater awareness of it and a lot of help is available for parents. It's not a disease that strikes at random; it's a condition that can occur because of particular circumstances and it's a condition that can be very successfully treated and prevented from recurring. It's also very common - as many as three or four children in a typical school class in the UK may be affected - so you can guarantee that you won't be the only parent seeking help.

Tackling child obesity early helps children lay the foundation stones for a healthy life and these are things they can pass on to their own children when they become parents. By helping your child, you will also be helping yourself to establish a healthy, active life that will benefit the whole family.

When writing this book, it really brought it home to me how children's lives have changed over the last couple of decades, and how easy it is for unhealthy habits to take over in what has been called an 'obesigenic environment'. I was also amazed at how much support and effort is going into solving the problem from all directions, which should be very encouraging for anyone who is worried about their children's weight.

Although this book often refers to 'your child', it is intended as a resource for anyone concerned with children's welfare, whether they are relatives, friends, teachers, childcare workers or professionals. It is not intended to replace professional advice but can be used as a handbook and reference guide to child obesity.

Disclaimer

This book is for general information on child obesity and weight issues, and is not intended to replace professional medical advice. It can be used alongside professional medical advice, but anyone thinking about introducing changes to their child's lifestyle, is strongly advised to consult their health care professional.

Chapter One

What Do We Mean by Obese?

A weighty problem

Obesity is a condition describing a child who is so seriously overweight for their age and height that their ability to take part in many childhood activities is affected. Even if it does not cause them any obvious medical problems at first, obese children are likely to be storing up serious health problems for the future.

Many people use the word 'obese' without really understanding that it is a precise medical term which doctors arrive at by measuring Body Mass Index (BMI). Calculating BMI involves comparing weight to height by dividing the weight measurement (in kilograms) by the square of the height (in meters). An adult with a BMI of over 30 would be considered obese.

Adult calculations are not suitable for children who are constantly growing and changing, and there is a lot of debate about the best ways to measure and define child obesity. The clinical definition of being overweight and obese for children is based on growth charts known as centile charts with different ones for boys and girls. These can be plotted and used with different cut off points in accordance with age and height. (See chapter 3 for more information on this.)

It's not necessary for a child to be officially stamped as 'obese' before any action needs to be taken. Considering that Foresight, a government sponsored project, has predicated that by 2050 a quarter of all Britain's children will be obese, it's in the interests of every parent to make sure that their child is not storing up problems for the future.

The future is fat

'A landmark report from a government sponsored project, Foresight, warned in 2007 that more than half of adults and a quarter of children will be dangerously overweight by 2050.'

It isn't only parents who are concerned about weight and obesity. It's a huge concern for governments, schools and the NHS, all of which are struggling to cope with the child obesity epidemic. The topic is never out of the media, and despite all of this interest, obesity rates are still on the rise and we're still heading for a fat future.

Some of the media attention is not helpful, particularly the constant focus on celebrity body shapes and diets. If parents are confused about whether their son or daughter is starving or stuffing themselves, imagine how children must feel when faced with a barrage of contradictions about body shape and size.

What are the facts?

According to the World Health Organisation there are ten facts that everyone needs to know about obesity.

1. Obesity has now reached epidemic levels in the UK.

2. Children especially are in danger of becoming obese.

3. Obesity is caused by not burning off more calories than you eat.

4. The cost of obesity to society is enormous.

5. Obesity tends to be more common in socially deprived communities.

6. Nobody is responsible for being overweight or obese.

7. Our eating habits have changed dramatically in the last few decades.

8. Most children and adults are not active enough.

9. Combating obesity requires healthy eating and increased physical activity.

10. There is a lot of support for people who need help in combating obesity.

These facts are worth looking at in detail to see how they apply to children.

1. The obesity 'epidemic'

An epidemic refers to an illness, disease or condition that is occurring on a much bigger scale than normal and is affecting a lot more people than would be expected.

The figures speak for themselves; the obesity charity Weight Concern estimates that 350,000 children in the UK are obese and at risk, and according to the World Health Organisation, rates in Europe have tripled in the last 20 years and by 2010 there will be 15 million obese children and adolescents.

In 2002, according to UK government health surveys, 22 per cent of boys and 28 per cent of girls aged 2 to 15 were either overweight or obese.

This high occurrence of obesity may help children to understand that they are far from unique and there are many others in the same situation.

2. Obesity danger for children

Children, especially in their early years, are very vulnerable and when it comes to eating they often have no control over the kind of food they are given. If they establish patterns of unhealthy eating choices in childhood, this is likely to stay with them throughout their lives.

In the first few years of life, a child's body lays down cells to store fat. The more fat that is stored, the larger the number of cells created, in order to store more fat. It's estimated that an obese child can have as many as three times the number of fat cells as a non-obese child, and when this process stops, the fat cells remain with the child for the rest of their life.

The amount of fat the body wants to store is in proportion to the number of cells that have been created. So if you were overweight as a child, the theory goes that your body is programmed to carry more fat. Although this stored fat can be lost by dieting or exercising, it is much more difficult to lose excess weight and better to try to avoid it. Put simply, you can prevent your child from suffering ill health in later life due to obesity - and for young children prevention is much better than the cure.

Most parents know about the importance of a balanced diet but it's your responsibility to safeguard your own child from future problems.

3. Don't eat more calories than you can burn off

This is a simple enough equation which children should be able to identify with.

4. Obesity is everybody's problem

It's not just individuals who suffer from the effects of obesity - it has a knock on effect for family members, friends, schools, the health service and society in general.

Obesity currently costs the NHS around £1 billion to treat each year, with an overall cost to the economy of up to £2.6 billion, and it has been suggested the future cost of treating the obesity epidemic could bankrupt the NHS.

Obese children are likely to be absent from school and underachieve. As employees, people who develop complications as a result of their weight will need to take more time off work and this will have an impact on their colleagues.

5. Obesity is linked to poverty and deprivation

According to the latest health surveys in England and Scotland, higher concentrations of obesity tend to be found in less well-off areas. If you look at the statistics on a map, you will see that there tends to be more cases of obesity in inner city areas. Some children will find themselves in a vicious circle of being obese because of social inequalities and being discriminated against because they are obese.

It is, however, important to note that any child from any background can become obese and the condition certainly isn't confined to one particular group of people in society.

6. It's not your fault

Another point to stress to children is that they should not be made to feel guilty about being overweight. The society we now live in has been described as an 'obesigenic environment', which actually increases the risk of becoming obese. This is down to the way modern society operates.

There's no single reason why obesity rates are so high, but a number of factors around food and lifestyle have combined to cause the current situation. Over a generation our lives have changed dramatically with fewer people doing heavy manual work and more people sitting in front of computers all day. At home we sit in front of screens watching a wide choice of TV channels or using a home computer. We have more money to spend on more types of food than ever before and although there is a huge interest in sport, it tends to be of the armchair variety. We generally travel by car and have houses packed full of gadgets and devices, which means we don't have to use much energy.

In this kind of atmosphere it is wrong to hold individuals responsible for their size and condition.

7. Too much food on the menu

The type of food we eat has changed almost as dramatically as our high-tech homes. We have a vast and tempting choice of different types of food every time we visit one of our well-stocked supermarkets. Many dishes are already prepared so we don't need to spend any energy cooking them.

Children are tempted by lots of brands and foods aimed at them specifically and it can be very difficult to resist pester power. Processed food, takeaways, ready meals and high energy drinks are bigger and more calorific than ever before – some burger meals can contain a child's entire calorific needs for the whole day.

Portion sizes have grown as food has become cheaper and children's spending power means that for a few pounds they can buy much bigger bars of chocolates and packets of sweets.

Of course it's great to have more choice and to be able to buy the things you want, but the current combination of too much of the wrong type of food and not enough exercise is a recipe for disaster.

8. The couch potato lives on

The term 'couch potato' has been around for quite a few years and although twenty years ago people had the most basic computer games and fewer TV channels, today there are a lot more to keep them firmly on the couch. While we are eating more food and more types of food, we are becoming less active.

Most children don't even walk to a bus stop but start and finish their school day in the car. Local shops are closing down, and parents often don't let their children walk to them alone because it's not safe. It's recommended that children should be involved in physical activity for 60 minutes a day. It doesn't have to be sport and it doesn't have to be all in one go.

9. Eat well and stay active

Doing these two things together is vital for success in combating obesity. If your child understands how important these two elements are, they will be on the way to success.

You should also stress to your child that it's not just their responsibility to make sure these two things are done. Schools, the health service, local councils and supermarkets all have an important role to play in ensuring they keep our children healthy by providing healthy food choices and opportunities to become more active.

Experts from the World Health Organisation recommend that healthy food options should be made cheaper and more widely available in shops and school canteens, and energy-dense foods and drinks should be restricted and replaced by better nutritional quality foods.

The also suggest that opportunities for physical activity in everyday life should be made available through school and workplace programmes. This action must be backed by the authorities and everyone involved in the food industry, local government, education and sport.

10. Help is at hand

This is good news for children and parents – it means that the obesity problem is being taken seriously by governments, schools, the health service, food providers and supermarkets who are all involved in efforts to combat the epidemic.

All the countries in Europe have made a commitment to work towards improving child obesity through increased exercise and healthy food choices.

There are lots of resources and places you can go for help and support, as well as information from all parts of the community. Once you find out what help, support and information is available, it should be much easier to make progress. (See the help list and chapter 9 for more information on this.)

Summing Up

- Obesity is nobody's fault but everyone's responsibility.
- Obesity is a serious medical condition – but can be tackled.
- Too much food and not enough exercise is a bad combination.
- Obesity has grown out of our changing lifestyle.
- Obesity is a very widespread problem but there is a lot of help available.

Chapter Two

The Causes and Effects of Obesity

Obesity is not always due to overeating and lack of exercise

Not all cases of weight gain or obesity in children are down to overeating and lack of exercise. Children's weight may go up and down for many reasons, for example if they are taking certain types of steroids.

There are also a number of rare conditions that can cause obesity such as Prader-Willi Syndrome, a genetic condition leading to overeating through excessive appetite. Similarly Hypothyroidism is a condition where the thyroid gland is under active and doesn't produce enough hormones to keep the body functioning properly, leading to slow metabolism and inevitable weight gain.

Is it all in the genes?

Some cases of obesity may be linked to genes, but that's not the whole story. Although obesity does seem to run through families, this could be because parents are passing on their own unhealthy habits to their children. If you know of obesity in your family, use this as an incentive to help your child avoid the same pitfalls. Obesity is one family heirloom that no one should have to inherit.

When does obesity start?

Obesity can occur at any age but often starts in the womb, which is why it's vital for pregnant women to eat well and avoid junk. There's no need to eat for two and the emphasis should be on quality, not quantity.

After birth the recommendation is to give a baby nothing but breast milk for six months. Breast milk is gourmet food for babies, containing everything they need to thrive and grow. There is a large amount of evidence that not only can breastfeeding protect a baby from many early infections and diseases, but it lowers the risk of your baby growing into an obese child.

Weaning is similarly important as it's at this stage that a child meets solids and varieties of food. This is the best time for setting good eating patterns, not only will you get your child off to a healthy start but you will give your child the habits of a lifetime. During infancy it's important to use the information, support and advice available from your health visitor or clinic on weaning and child nutrition.

We all want the best for our children and go to a lot of effort and expense to give them the best we can and keep them safe from danger. Few parents would willingly neglect their children and leave them at risk, but children who grow up with unhealthy eating habits and inactive lifestyles are at risk from obesity, which can be so bad as to be life threatening. Most parents, family members and carers are simply not aware of the risks of obesity and it's worth examining some of the immediate and longer term health risks in detail.

Doctors have known for a long time that obese children are at risk of developing a number of conditions later in life, including heart disease, some cancers and osteoarthritis. However, in recent years, as the rates of obesity in the UK have soared, some diseases which had been considered the diseases of old age, have been occurring more in children - some as young as seven, which is a graphic indication of how serious the problem is.

Effects of obesity can last a lifetime

Obese children run the risk of becoming obese adults - more than 70% of obese children and more than 85% of obese adolescents will become obese adults.

For obese adolescents and young adults there is increased risk of doing badly in school, earning less and being excluded from friendship groups. Ultimately the effect of child obesity is an increased risk of ill health and premature death in adult life.

Short term - not just a cosmetic problem

In our size zero obsessed society it's easy to forget that being overweight isn't just about appearing to be fat. Children focus particularly on the cosmetic side of obesity, but losing weight is about more than trying to look good, it's about being healthy and fit for life.

Apart from looking fat, your child will also look unhealthy if they are missing out on vitamins and nutrients. Your child may be pale, spotty, have dry skin patches, suffer chafing or develop fungal infections under folds of skin. Too much sugar in their diet can rot teeth. Children on a poor diet are likely to suffer a sluggish digestion and may be constipated. They may have greasy hair and bad breath, all of which are difficult for children to cope with.

Long term - heart disease and stroke

Overweight children are likely to have high blood pressure, and in the long term this puts them at risk of heart disease and stroke. An unhealthy diet is also likely to contain very high levels of cholesterol, which will add to the problems.

The processes that lead to cardiovascular disease in later life are strongly associated with child obesity. Cardiovascular risk factors in obese children include raised blood lipids (fats), insulin levels and high blood pressure.

Approximately two thirds of children of primary school age who are obese will have at least one cardiovascular risk factor and approximately one quarter will have two or more. Although recent years have seen successes in cutting the number of deaths from heart disease, cardiologists fear the good work will be undone if obesity is not brought under control.

Type 2 Diabetes

Type 2 diabetes occurs when the amount of insulin produced by the body is inefficient or insufficient and does not work properly. In most cases this is linked with being overweight. Children as young as seven have recently been diagnosed with this disease.

According to Diabetes UK, this sort of diabetes, which is usually associated with middle age, has been observed in the USA for some time, and now in the UK there are estimated to be around 1000 children with Type 2 diabetes. These children are all clinically obese and face potential blindness, heart disease and amputations.

For more information see *Diabetes – The Essential Guide*.

Asthma

Child obesity is also associated with increased risk of asthma, and can make a child's existing asthma worse. One of the most important things for children with asthma is keeping fit and healthy, which they are encouraged to do. However, obese asthmatic children may not be able to do this.

Sleep apnoea

This is a sleeping disorder caused by a lack of oxygen in the blood while sleeping. It causes the sleeper to wake suddenly and may make them a heavy snorer. Sleep apnoea is closely linked to being overweight.

'It is estimated that there are around 1,000 children with Type 2 diabetes in the UK, all of whom are clinically obese. This means that there is a generation of overweight youngsters facing potential blindness, heart disease and amputations.'

Simon O'Neill, Director of Care, Information and Advocacy at Diabetes UK, speaking about the Foresight report in October 2007.

Cancer

Being very overweight increases the risk of cancer of the womb, kidney, colon, gallbladder and oesophagus (food pipe). Cancer Research UK suggests that in the UK, 12 thousand people could avoid getting cancer by not being overweight.

Osteoarthritis

Being overweight can put a tremendous strain on the joints, causing wear and tear beyond their years. Obese children may find their knees and hip joints ache under the pressure of carrying around so much excess weight. If the extra weight is taken off their joints in time, the damage will be reversed. But the longer it goes on, the more difficult it will be for a child to return to full health.

Psychological effects of being overweight

Doctors can diagnose and treat many of the illnesses that are caused by obesity, but one of the most difficult aspects to understand and treat is the psychological effect.

Children like to join in and belong, but an obese child may be excluded from many of the physical activities that children take for granted. Many playground games may be off limits for overweight children and being excluded will make matters worse through lack of exercise. Younger children will find themselves in a vicious circle - they may want to join in with sport and games, but won't be able to and won't get any benefit from activity and exercise.

Children, even at very early ages, are aware of the negative view society has towards obese people and it seems likely that this may influence their developing sense of self and self-esteem.

For obese adolescents, particularly girls, the consequences of being obese are worse and can lead to poor self-image. Teenage girls are much less likely than boys to get involved, or have opportunities to get involved, in physical activity, and even schools struggle to provide them with opportunities to keep active.

'It's difficult to measure the distress that negative attitudes can cause a child and they are perhaps worse than the physical reality of being overweight, as the scar is likely to remain with the child for many years.'

Again, the vicious circle of obesity being caused by lack of exercise, and the inability to exercise contributing to obesity, will kick in. Going into the teenage years is dangerous for obese adolescents on two scores. Not only will they have to deal with the emotional upheaval but they will have to do this as obese young people, giving them a whole different set of negative body images to contend with. Statistically they are also less likely to be able to combat their condition.

Survey of attitudes about obese children

In 1961 an American study into the stigmatisation of obese children, 'Cultural Uniformity in Reaction to Physical Disabilities', revealed how deep the negative images of overweight children really are. Primary school children were shown pictures of children with various kinds of disabilities and were asked to rank who they would like to be friends with, from first to last. The study found that every child said the person they would least like to be friends with was the obese child.

It is tempting to think that attitudes have changed since 1961, but when another team did a follow up in 2001, with the obesity rate doubled, they found that children's attitudes had changed for the worse and the same prejudices were still firmly in place.

Lack of chances in life

A British Medical Association report into obese children's life chances found evidence that obese children are more likely to suffer discrimination in life because of their condition and will be at increased risk of discrimination.

The good news about obesity

All this makes for very depressing reading but there is some good news about obesity. The fact is that children don't have to face a lifetime of devastating diseases and health complaints. Virtually all the complications caused by obesity in young children and adolescents, can be undone by taking simple actions.

'Girls with obesity are less likely to be accepted into university, and less likely to be married and be economically 'well off' in adulthood. Being overweight or obese is also more likely to have a negative impact on life satisfaction, and the future life of young women in particular, as girls are judged on body shape more than boys.'

BMA report: 'Preventing Childhood Obesity', 2005. www.bma.org.

Obesity is not a disease your child can catch in the same way as measles or mumps and it is likely to have been building up for a long time, for months or possibly years before it reaches a point where it can't be ignored. There's also no reason why children of obese parents should follow suit if they are able to act early enough to deal with the condition.

The younger you can start to tackle obesity in a child, the easier it is to beat it. A child below the age of 10 will stand a much better chance of losing weight quickly than an adolescent who may find it more difficult and is likely to grow into adulthood as obese if action isn't taken. Although prevention is always better than a cure, acting sooner rather than later will ensure you can halt or prevent all the major conditions associated with obesity.

Summing Up

- Obesity is a serious and possibly life threatening condition.
- It can be the cause of long term health problems.
- More children than ever are experiencing complications earlier.
- Most of the complications caused by obesity can be halted or reversed.

Chapter Three

Is My Child Overweight or Obese?

How can I tell?

Most parents don't know if their child is obese. Eating habits, mealtimes, portion sizes and the type of food we eat have all changed so much that it's impossible to say anymore what makes up three square meals a day.

Children are also getting bigger and taller than previous generations; add to this the fact that their body shape is constantly changing and you can see how difficult it can be for parents to form an accurate view of their child's weight.

In 2007, when a research team led by the Department of Epidemiology and Public Health at University College London, asked parents in outer London to describe their child's weight, they found some very confused views about obesity. Only six per cent of parents with obese or overweight children in the early years of primary school described their child as overweight. The same pattern occurred in the older age groups too.

Researchers concluded that most parents of overweight children are just not switched on to how severe their child's condition is and have no idea of what a healthy child looks like.

The same study suggests that parents' views of acceptable eating habits are based on what their friends and neighbours do, so if the family across the road eat ready meals, and fast food and drink lots of fizzy drinks, then it can't be that bad.

'Researchers at UCL found that among 500 children in nursery and reception classes in the outer London area, only six per cent of parents with overweight or obese children described their child as overweight.'

The problem with this sort of thinking is that not all children are equally active and it can result in obesity if parents don't make sure their child does enough exercise to burn off the junk.

Some parents may also believe that if their child is labelled 'obese' it will reflect badly on them and their lifestyle. The biggest challenge for some families may be to accept that they will only be able to help their child if they try to change some of their habits.

Are you in denial?

Parental denial can be a big obstacle to tackling a weight problem in children. Not only is this a problem for their children, but also for teachers or carers who may be concerned.

It's easy for adults to notice changes to their own body size and shape but it's much more difficult to understand what changing shapes mean for children. Puppy fat or chubby cheeks may be part of your child's body gearing up for a growth spurt. Look through old photos and see how your child's face shape changes over a matter of months and you will see how much of a variation there can be.

Many parents will also be in denial because admitting their child has unhealthy habits means they will be forced to examine their own lifestyles. Sometimes it's just easier to stay the way you are and not to rock the boat.

Weighing it all up

There are many ways you can check and track your child's weight, either by yourself or with the help of your health care team. There's a lot of debate about which method might be best but here are some of the main options for monitoring weight.

Body Mass Index (BMI)

We looked at BMI or Body Mass Index in chapter 1. It's a way of assessing whether someone's weight is putting their health at risk. It is calculated by dividing weight in kilograms by height in meters squared.

Although a child's BMI is calculated in the same way as an adult's would be, adult figures must not be used for children and there are special age and gender specific charts available like the ones below. These are called centile charts and are plotted to give cut off points, which give a definition of obesity.

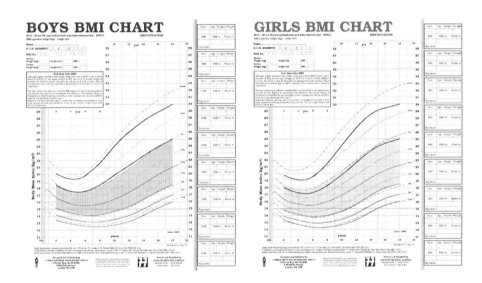

© Child Growth Foundation

Doctors define obese children as those with a BMI over the 98th centile of the UK 1990 reference chart for age and sex. Overweight children are defined as those with a BMI above the 91st centile. BMI is not a failsafe way of calculating whether your child is overweight and results should be interpreted by a health care professional.

You can do most things online these days and calculating your child's BMI is no exception. The charity Weight Concern has a calculator for children you can use. Notice how important your child's date of birth and the current date are in the calculation - this reflects the rate at which children grow and change.

Waist to height ratio

Rather than focus on a child's weight there is a way recommended by the website www.weightlossresources.co.uk, which allows you to monitor a child's size as they grow, without using scales.

To do this, measure your child's height and waist circumference, then divide the waist measurement by the height measurement. For example, for a child who has a waist circumference of 55 cm and is 122 cm tall, the calculation is $55 \div 122 = 0.45$.

A cut off point of 0.5 should be used to indicate potential weight problems – in other words, where the waist measurement is half the height measurement. Children who have a waist to height ratio of more than 0.5 are likely to be overweight – and the larger the number, the greater the potential problem.

Speaking to health professionals

Although DIY weighing, measuring and monitoring may give you a good idea about your child's weight, it's important not to set too much store by the results without consulting a health professional. This could be your doctor, a health visitor, practice nurse or your pharmacist. They will be able to offer advice, reassurance and talk you through the options available. After you start on a programme of healthy eating, you can use your favourite method of weighing or measuring to track your child's progress.

Speaking to your child

We will look later at talking to your child but it's important to consider their feelings before you start sizing them up. Some children are interested in their weight but it's important not to make a big issue of this before you start.

Why are some schools weighing and measuring children?

Children in the reception and final year of primary school in England and Wales are now having their weight and height measured in school on a voluntary basis. This is for government statistics on children's health. The results are available to parents on request and there has been recent talk about sending out warning letters to parents if their child is found to be excessively overweight. It's up to you whether to get involved in this programme but it might be helpful to tap into the resources the school should be able to offer you.

Children at risk

Even if your child doesn't hit the overweight or obesity cut off points, there are certain things which could make them prone to obesity in the future:

- Spending more than two hours a day in front of a TV or computer.
- Not fitting into clothes for their age, especially round the waist.
- Not being interested in activity and getting puffed out easily.
- Bingeing on certain foods and having excessive faddy eating habits.
- Eating lots of crisps, biscuits, sweets, chocolate and high fat foods.
- Spending less than 30 minutes a day being active.
- Parents or siblings being obese.
- Picking their own food.
- Eating less than five portions of fruit and vegetables a day.
- Eating in front of the TV.

'Try talking to your local pharmacy - they will be able to offer free confidential advice, information and support and there's sure to be one near you.'

Ethnic risk groups

Children from some ethnic groups need to be particularly careful about unwanted weight gain. Surveys from the British Heart Foundation report, 'Couch Kids – the Continuing Epidemic', show that girls from the Pakistani and Afro Caribbean community are more at risk of developing obesity, while boys from the Indian and Pakistani community are at risk of being overweight. In general children from all South Asian communities are four times as likely to be obese than children from the white population, and they are also less likely to have the chance to exercise.

Development of obesity

You won't wake up one morning to find your child has grown like the Incredible Hulk; the problem will have been building up for months, if not years, as a result of a long standing, unhealthy eating and couch potato lifestyle. Excess weight will not vanish overnight and it will take time to make changes which achieve results, so it's important for you to start with a positive attitude to help carry your child through.

What is a healthy weight?

Guessing a child's healthy weight is a bit like trying to pin the tail on the donkey. Even if you get it right, your answer may only be valid for a couple of months or even weeks as your child will quickly outgrow the answer. A healthy weight is one which is appropriate for your child's age and is part of a healthy lifestyle. A child with a healthy weight will be able to be active without being impeded by their size, will have a healthy appetite and will generally feel and look well.

If you're still not sure about this, speak to your family doctor or practice nurse who will reassure you. Don't listen to Grandma, friends, neighbours or work colleagues - they may be well intentioned, but they too are trying to pin the tail on the donkey.

Nobody's fault, everybody's responsibility

It's important to avoid blaming anyone for your child's health, especially your child. Although we can all certainly do better to help our children, there's no point in blaming Grandma for giving your child too many sweets. A toddler who is only offered nuggets and chips at children's parties can't really do much to choose a healthy option. A teenager who eats chips for lunch at a college canteen where they only serve chips, is only making things worse. The boy who avoids exercise at school because they only play team games, for which he never gets chosen, can't be held responsible for not getting enough exercise.

If your child can't eat lunch because the school doesn't have a proper dining room and the children are eating at their desks due to overcrowding, it's not their fault. Your child is the way they are because they have grown up in a less than ideal situation - the 'obesigenic environment'. However, your child is lucky because with the right understanding and attitude, you can help them change life for the better.

Summing Up

- Get the facts from an expert about your child's weight.

- If your child is not obese, make sure they don't get that way.

- Measuring children can be useful but is only one part of keeping healthy.

- There is no such thing as an ideal weight for children, only a healthy lifestyle.

Try the fun quiz at the back of this book (Appendix A) to see how healthy your family is.

Chapter Four

Getting Ready to Tackle Obesity

We've looked at some of the facts and the background to obesity, so you should have an understanding of why it's important to get your child on track for a healthy lifestyle. You may have tried to change your child's eating habits in the past or thought vaguely that they could be overweight. You both may have wanted to do something about it, but there always seems to be a good reason not to. Now it's time to take action!

The energy imbalance

Let's remind ourselves of the main reason for unwanted weight gain - the energy imbalance. It sounds very simple: if you take in more energy than you use, you will put on weight. The solution is also simple, take in less energy and burn more off. In practical terms this might not mean eating less, but just eating less of certain types of food and using up more energy in physical activity and exercise.

Don't gain, maintain

One important point about children is that unlike adults, they may not actually need to lose weight to be healthy. Growing children generally have a higher metabolic rate compared to adults, and active children have an even higher metabolic rate. The trick is to stop gaining and start maintaining weight by balanced eating and activity - this way most children should be able to continue to grow healthily and avoid unnecessary weight gain.

Surgical and medical options

So far we've concentrated on lifestyle changes in the battle against obesity, but there are some options available for the most severe forms of obesity. These include stomach stapling, gastric banding and drugs.

Using surgery and adult drugs to treat obesity in children is risky and controversial, with unknown consequences. These are not methods to take lightly and are a last resort, which will require expert medical advice and support every step of the way. The first step to using these would be a consultation with your GP.

No quick fixes in getting fit for life

There are no miracle cures or quick fixes, but once you have enough information and support, you can work a bit of magic in transforming your child's life by committing yourselves to a healthier lifestyle.

Everyone has seen television programmes that take an overweight, unhealthy person and turn his or her life around. At 7pm we will meet the 'star', a desperate man or woman undergoing this week's makeover. By 7.30pm we are presented with a totally new and transformed person, two stones lighter, with a new wardrobe, a new haircut and a new life.

Even though the transformation is genuine, it's not as simple as it looks. Behind the scenes there will have been a small army of people working away to make this possible. The 'star' will have spent weeks, if not months, following a strict schedule devised by expert dieticians, doctors, life coaches and fitness trainers. There is also the added motivation of not wanting to fail in front of millions of viewers!

You might not have a team of experts at your disposal but you will have support, and you may live in an area where they run a special programme for children. Find out what's available and access as much support as you can. Be aware though that it's you and your child who will need to work hard on kicking bad habits and replacing them with healthy patterns of behaviour.

Talking to your child

All parents want the best for their children and if your son or daughter is already keen to make changes, so much the better. If you're making the decision to do something for your child, then you need to think carefully about how you're going to talk to them about it. People involved in childcare and education will also need to think carefully about how they want to approach the subject in conjunction with a child's parents. The following advice should be helpful for everyone.

Think about how much you want to say to your child and what you expect them to do about it. Bear in mind, and stress to your child if they are old enough, that the situation of being overweight isn't anybody's fault, but it's not doing anybody any good and it won't go away without your whole family making some changes.

Younger children

All children need healthy eating and activity messages, but for younger children action is probably more important than words. It's also easier to get under fives eating healthily as you have more control over what they eat. Follow advice from your health visitor and teach them the basics of five a day, a balanced diet and healthy snacking. Also try to get your child to participate in some form of activity everyday.

Older children

Between the ages of 7 and 11, children have more choice about what they eat so you will need their cooperation and understanding if you want them to make changes to eating habits - but you still need to do a lot of the thinking and decision making for them.

From 12 onwards, adolescents will have more understanding about food, weight and body shape, although their knowledge might not be from the best available sources. They should be able to come up with ideas to help themselves and you will need to let them make their own decisions about healthy eating and activity.

Broaching the subject

If your child brings up the subject let them talk and see how far it takes you. If the conversation turns to making plans then you can progress to that stage.

'Parents can be uneasy about raising the issue of overweight, fearing that to do so will hurt their child's feelings. Like all sensitive issues, there are more and less helpful ways of talking to your child about their weight.'
Weight Concern.
www.weightconcern.co.uk

If you need to start a conversation with your child about their weight, you could bring up the subject by asking how they feel when:

- other people comment about their size.
- buying clothes that are for older age groups.
- they are teased about their size.
- they are not able to get involved in sports and games.

You could ask if this kind of thing upsets them and if they would like you to help them do something about it. If you know someone who has been in a similar situation point this out and use them as a good example.

It's vital to talk

Not dealing with obesity and the issue of being overweight, however difficult it may be to start a conversation, means the problem will not go away and your child might try risky dieting, which could be more dangerous than doing nothing.

What to avoid and what to emphasise

Here are some helpful pieces of advice from the charity Weight Concern.

When talking to your child about their weight:

✓	✗
Tell them that you recognise how hard it is to make healthy choices.	Don't tell your child that they're 'greedy' or 'lazy'.
Praise them when you see them eating healthily.	Don't make your child feel guilty about their eating habits.
Ask them what would be good about being less heavy.	Don't scare your child into trying to lose weight.
Ask them about what action they think would help.	Don't moan about your own weight and how 'boring' being on a diet is.

Thinking about yourself and setting a good example

Parents and carers are the most important role models for children and young people, and your attitudes and approaches can have a positive influence on children. If you sit on the sofa eating a donut and attempt to tell your child about the importance of healthy living, they may see right through you. If you always drive to school or use the car on short trips to the shops, then think about how that might look to your child if you're trying to get them to walk more.

The important thing is to lead by example and you may have to re-think your own habits before trying to change your child's. It would also be helpful when talking about the issues of being overweight and obese, to think about whether you could help your child by following some of these pieces of advice:

- Don't make negative comments about overweight people - you don't know why they are the way they are.

- Point out that no one is perfect and everyone has good points and attractive features.

- Don't let your child believe that there is an ideal weight for them, and that they will only be happy if they reach this weight.

- Tell your child that it can be difficult for some people to control their weight but the main thing is to have healthy habits.

The word 'diet'

You may have noticed the 'd' word is mostly absent from this book and when it does pop up, it's used to mean eating patterns in general and not the sort of thing that people spend years trying and failing to do.

Dieting and slimming are two words being left off the menu because they are not really helpful to obese or overweight children. A diet is a temporary eating plan which may cause some loss of weight because it generally excludes certain groups of foods. Children don't need to do this and it's harmful for a growing child to start cutting out food groups from their daily intake.

Obese children don't need to 'slim down' to an 'ideal weight', and even if there was an ideal average weight for their size, it probably wouldn't remain that way for very long. Your child should understand that you are not aiming to arrive at a 'perfect' weight but to stabilise and maintain weight through healthy eating and activity.

Healthy choices should be easy choices

Prevention of child obesity involves the child, family, school, the health services, and the community. A child can't be held responsible for giving in to the temptation to binge and gorge on unhealthy stuff when there's so much of it around and it's so easily available. Healthy choices should be easy choices to make and unless everyone involved in caring for children supports this and provides options concerning food and activity, the only choices available could be unhealthy.

A family affair

Most of the evidence about successful weight control points to the fact that children who have the support of their families are more motivated and more successful. Since families tend to reinforce bad eating habits and sedentary lifestyles, it's logical that they can make good habits acceptable. While it might be unrealistic to expect siblings to give up their favourite sweets or treats, everyone in the family should start thinking about choosing healthier options or at least keeping their bad habits to themselves for a while.

All of the immediate family do need to be on board and understand what you're trying to achieve because it won't work if anyone in the family makes fun or won't join in. It might be worth taking family members aside and speaking to them about the consequences of not getting eating habits under control if they don't support you. It's also a good idea to ask grandparents, aunties and uncles to cut back on the treats they give your child, or replace them with toys, magazines or healthy options.

Motivation and self-esteem

Changing the habits of a lifetime is never easy, as anyone who has abandoned their New Year's resolutions on January 2nd will tell you. The changes an obese child needs to make will bring about a massive, life long improvement. Once the realisation of this kicks in later down the line, your child will get a big sense of achievement, which should give them the confidence to go on and tackle new challenges.

In the short term, it will be difficult but it's important to keep motivation and morale high. You could give your child small incentives along the way, which will also help to mark progress and make them feel better about themselves. These could be things like a new haircut, or some clothes - things that your child can use to improve their appearance.

Notice the good things about your child

Boosting a child's self esteem will give them the motivation and confidence to move forward through the difficult early days. Tell your child when you notice things you like about them, eg a nice smile, a funny joke, a kind thought. Find something your child is good at and can concentrate on aside from beating obesity. Above all, let your child know that they are loved and appreciated and that you're working though this process with them.

You might want to put together a scrap book of your child's achievements over the years, certificates, school reports and old pictures and show it to them so they can see and value their past achievements.

'All of the immediate family really do need to be on board and understand what you're trying to achieve because it won't work if anyone in the family makes fun or won't join in.'

Summing Up

- There are no easy options to weight loss.
- Your child is not going on a diet.
- Take some time to talk to your child.
- Get the family on board.
- Make sure your child feels valued and appreciated.

Chapter Five

Small Steps to Success

Obesity is everyone's problem

Just as no child is responsible for being obese, no child should be responsible for sorting it out alone. A lot of the organisations which children come into contact with have long been aware of the obesity time bomb and are doing their utmost to help.

Sources of help

Schools have been criticised for not doing enough to promote healthy eating to children, but some schools have been working hard to bring about changes for a long time. Supermarkets are also on the case and have lots of information for parents and children with weight control in mind – often they have special ranges for children or low fat food selections.

Your local council also has a role to play and should be able to help you find some fun leisure activities. They also have a responsibility to improve cycle and walking routes around your child's school and where you live.

Let's take a more detailed look at what sort of things these organisations might be able to do for you and what you can expect from them.

Nurseries and playgroups

All places that care for children should take an interest in their health and well-being and there's no better place to start than playgroup or nursery. If your child attends or is going to attend any sort of pre-school care, here are some key questions to ask:

- Are healthy snacks available?

- Are the children given plain water or fruit juice?

- How active are the children - do they have regular physical activities, are they taken outdoors, do they have space to move around inside?

- Do the children learn about healthy eating, which foods are good and which to avoid?

'Hungry for Success is a whole school approach to educating young people about healthy eating. The aim is to break the culture of unhealthy eating in Scotland so that children and young people will opt for healthier food, not only in school but also outside of school.'

What can your school do?

Just as our eating habits at home have changed in the last couple of decades, so have school canteens. No more eating under the beady eye of the teacher - most schools are self-service with a varied menu and the rise of the lunch box means children can be more picky about what they eat.

In Scotland, a scheme called Hungry for Success was launched in 2003 to improve school meals in all Scottish schools. Hungry for Success was recognised by Jamie Oliver for being ahead of its time in the UK.

Most schools are also striving to play their part in making sure children get their recommended 60 minutes a day of activity and there are wide variations in what's on offer in different parts of the country.

Opposite are some questions you might want to ask your child's school, and key points that schools should consider.

Your local council

Councils are responsible for many areas which impact on children's lives - not in the least schools. Councils provide and licence many services that a child will use, ranging from day nurseries, playgroups, activity clubs, after school clubs and many sport facilities. They maintain cycle paths, parks and leisure facilities, provide public transport and sports centres.

Find out if there are any special programmes or activities for overweight children, that you can do as a family. It doesn't have to be the treadmill at the local gym, it could be rock climbing, skiing, skating, or sailing - the list is endless!

Primary School	Secondary School
How do you get healthy eating and exercise messages across to children?	How are healthy lifestyles promoted in the school?
Do you provide special low fat menus for children trying to control their weight?	Is the school making any effort to ensure that healthy options are available at lunchtime and that children choose them?
Where do the children eat their lunch and how is lunchtime organised?	Are the children allowed to go out of school for their lunch and if so how does that square with healthy eating?
Are there any rules about lunch boxes, are chocolate bars and sweets allowed?	Does the school have vending machines selling fizzy drinks and confectionery, and do they have control of the contents?
How do you encourage the children to play actively in the playground?	What efforts are being made to actively encourage children with weight issues to get involved in sporting activities?
What facilities do you have for PE, and how do you manage obese children?	Are there any extra activities suitable for overweight children either at lunchtime or after school?
Does the school promote walking to school or have a 'walking bus'?	How does the school cover healthy eating in home economics?
Are there any after school activities my child could join in with?	Is there any agreed strategy in the local education authority area for tackling obesity?

Councils have responsibility for making sure streets and cycle paths are safe and clean for children to use. It's also been suggested that councils could do more by working with local shops and businesses to promote healthy choices and should make sure that all food available in cafés that come under their jurisdiction complies with healthy living.

In Scotland, Wales and Northern Ireland the devolved governments and assemblies are very active in promoting healthy living and there are some very imaginative schemes and initiatives going on. If you live in one of these parts of the UK then it's worth contacting the relevant health department to find out about more localised support.

Your local health board

From your local health centre you should be able to access support from your GP, practice nurse and health visitor. If necessary, they will be able to refer you to other services within your local health board area, in order for you to get more help. Your local pharmacy will also be able to give advice and support and may be worth a visit. Information is generally available in different languages and formats. These groups should be able to:

'Don't forget at election time when the politicians are in hot pursuit of your vote, to quiz them about what they are doing to encourage healthy lifestyles among children in their locality. If you think they should be doing more, tell them!'

- Provide help and advice on a long term basis.
- Tell you about the benefits of healthy living.
- Have a range of suggestions about how to keep your child active.
- Come up with some healthy eating suggestions for children.
- Help you set some goals for your child.
- Give advice on various options and offer useful contacts.

Web

I've included some useful websites and contact details in the final chapter but it's worth spending a bit of time surfing for your own sites. Make a special folder in your bookmarks and subscribe to feeds to keep yourself updated. Visit parenting sites and join forums where you can exchange experiences and ideas. It's free and anonymous and you're sure to be able to pick up some useful tips.

If you are looking for more specialised advice, for example if you belong to a particular ethnic group or if you have special dietary requirements, then you might be able to find helpful information.

Time for change

If you and your child are ready to start making changes to your lifestyles, you might want to spend some time thinking about what you're aiming for and planning for success. Talk about what you think might work and what might not be useful. Every child is different and they will want more of some things and less of others, so be flexible and decide what you can achieve.

Food and Activity Diary (FAD) - Appendix B

Start by getting your child to keep a Food and Activity Diary (FAD), like the one in Appendix B. Do this honestly for a week and write down everything your child eats and all forms of activity, exercise or sport they take part in. This can be school PE, swimming, walking to school or even playing.

If your child dislikes the idea of form filling, you could do this as a video diary - as long as it's honest and covers all eating and activity. A camcorder diary has the added advantage that your child will be able to see how much they have changed over the weeks.

Food and Activity Plan (FAP) - Appendix C

Pick a week when your child wants to start being more healthy and active. Using the information on your child's FAD, start to think about what you might be able to change. Write these things down on the Food and Activity Plan (FAP).

Aim for some easily achievable swaps and substitutions in the first week – you might want to swap a couple of fizzy drinks for fresh juice, or a chocolate bar for a bunch of grapes. Make sure you include some activity, whether it's walking to school or bouncing on the trampoline.

You might want to include weight, BMI and waist circumference on the FAP to chart your child's progress. However, don't put too much importance on this in the early days or over stress the weight loss element.

'The most successful attempts at weight management start with small incremental steps which slowly build up on each other towards successful weight maintenance.'

Laura Stewart, Dietician.

www.childrensweightclinic.com

Use the charts on the FAP to record what your child eats and does during the first week of making healthy choices. The chart lets you give your child points for each positive choice made and you can add this up at the end of each week to give them a 'personal best'. Fill in the FAP everyday and then repeat the process at the end of every week. You can continue with this for as long as is necessary.

You should be able to notice more positive changes the longer it goes on month by month. It's also a good idea to include how your child is feeling and any changes they may notice – feeling less tired, feeling fitter, having more energy, clearer skin - as this will show the benefits of the new lifestyle.

Recognising achievements with rewards

Motivation is important to get your child up and running, so when they do start to make progress, it's important to make them aware that you recognise this. When you see your child making healthy choices let them know how pleased you are. If your child gets lots of points on the action plan, reward this with a small present. It could be an item of clothing, small toy, or a magazine.

By doing this, you are letting your child know how well they are progressing and you are breaking the connection between unhealthy treats like sweets being seen as rewards for good behaviour. Try not to use the rewards as bribes, 'if you eat that broccoli I'll give you a new set of pens' - keep the rewards as a surprise instead.

Summing Up

- Find out what support is out there and make the most of it.

- Keep the FAD as honestly as possible.

- Plan for success with your FAP, but be realistic about what you can achieve.

- Make sure all the places where your child spends time are sympathetic to their needs.

- Make sure you recognise and reward your child's attempts at being healthy.

Chapter Six
The Basics of
Healthy Eating

Back to basics

Every five-year-old knows how many portions of fruit and vegetables they should eat everyday, yet, although most of us understand this healthy eating message, putting it into practice isn't always that simple.

Much has been written about children and their food – enough to fill a whole book on the subject - but if you understand the basics you can easily start to make the small changes that lead to success.

Most young children have strong opinions about food, and older children in particular will have quite sophisticated tastes. We know a lot more about exotic dishes and have a much bigger choice than ever before, but we seem to have lost an understanding of the very basics of food and healthy eating.

It's worthwhile looking at some basic facts about food, before thinking about what to do with it.

Healthy eating on a plate

The picture on the next page shows how food can be split into groups and what proportions they should be served in. If you get the proportions right, you'll be on your way to establishing a very basic but important mealtime eating pattern.

Healthy Food Plate

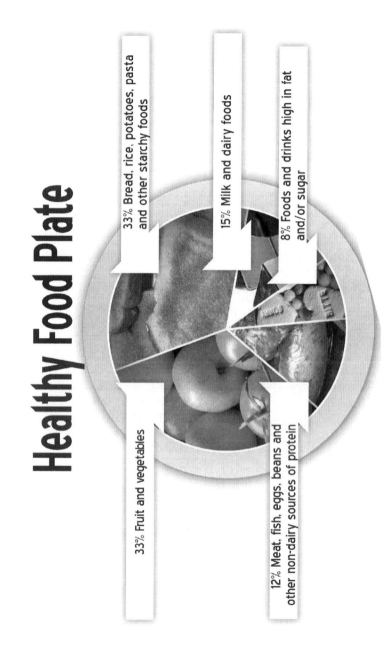

33% Bread, rice, potatoes, pasta and other starchy foods

15% Milk and dairy foods

8% Foods and drinks high in fat and/or sugar

33% Fruit and vegetables

12% Meat, fish, eggs, beans and other non-dairy sources of protein

Percentages used are those recommended by the Food Standards Agency.
www.food.gov.uk

Balancing act

Healthy eating depends on balancing types of food in the right proportions to give children the right mix in the right amounts. Each food group is important for children and none should be left out entirely.

Food groups for thought

Starchy foods

These are things like bread, cereal, potatoes, rice and pasta - foods that keep energy levels up through the day. Although they are not fattening in themselves, the spreads and sauces that often go with them can be.

Fruit and vegetables

These contain fibre and vitamins and are vital in helping to control weight. Fresh, frozen, tinned or dried fruit and vegetables all count towards your five a day, as do smoothies and fresh juice.

Meat, fish or vegetarian alternatives

These contain protein for growth and energy. Eggs, beans, lentils and tofu are vegetarian and low fat alternatives. Children should eat oily fish such as tuna and mackerel once or twice a week.

Milk and dairy

Milk and cheese contain calcium, which is vital for children and teenagers with growing bones. Under twos should have full-fat varieties but older children should use skimmed or semi-skimmed milk.

Sugar and fat

Fats are important for health but many types of ready meals, snacks and biscuits contain excessive amounts, particularly of nasty things called trans fats. Sugar is not forbidden but is so common now that we take much more than we need. Your child will need to cut right back on these to get their weight under control.

Drink

Children should have up to eight glasses of water a day to keep themselves hydrated. Also to save young teeth, restrict juice to mealtimes. Fizzy drinks should be left out or cut back as much as possible.

'Cooking skills are definitely a big thing. We've almost got a generation who lack basic cooking skills and don't know about things that are quick and nice and easy to make.'

Laura Stewart, Dietician,

www.childrensweightclinic.com

How to use food groups

Now that we've looked at food groups, here's some tips to help you use them:

- Base meals around starchy foods such as potatoes, bread, rice and pasta, but avoid brown rice and brown pasta for the under fives.

- Make the most of foods with plenty of fibre, such as fruit and vegetables, oats, grains, seeds, beans, peas and lentils.

- The five a day message is a minimum recommendation, aim for more.

- Avoid high sugar and high fat foods, deep fried foods and takeaway pies and pastries which may contain excessive amounts of fat and sugar.

- Choose low fat varieties of milk and dairy products where possible but watch for artificial sugars in yoghurts.

- Try to choose low fat versions of burgers and sausages, and grill or barbecue rather than fry.

- Make your own burgers and nuggets (see recipes in chapter 7). Your children will love them and at least you'll know what's in them.

- Eat a healthy breakfast everyday, cereal is fine but should be low sugar and accompanied by a portion of fruit.

- Watch portion sizes and avoid overloading plates with too much of any one type of food - aim for variety.

■ Cut back on ketchup and sauces - you may use these to add taste but they are also adding sugar and additives.

Can't cook, won't cook?

Although many people take an interest in cookery programmes and food, their skills in the kitchen are often limited to programming the microwave. Basic cookery need not be time consuming. Cooking for your family is much more rewarding, definitely healthier and probably cheaper than the alternatives.

Dietician Laura Stewart, who runs a weight loss clinic for children in Edinburgh, suggests that lack of cookery skills could be a big hurdle to eating healthily and if we are to beat the obesity epidemic, we need to know how to do it.

It's worth brushing up on your cookery skills - find out if there are any evening courses in your area that you could do with an older child. You're not aiming to be a top chef, but once you've mastered the basics you'll be more confident and will have a much more varied menu. If you can't do a course, get a basic cookery book; Delia Smith and Jamie Oliver have both written books for people starting from scratch.

Get the whole family involved in cooking their meals and have competitions to see who can make the most popular dish in the family.

'Get the whole family involved in cooking their meals and have competitions to see who can make the most popular dish in the family.'

Get a feel for food

Try getting back to basics with food and finding out where you can get fresh produce in your area. Look out for farmers' markets, independent shops, farm shops, or pick your own. You could find out if it's possible to have a bag of fresh seasonal fruit and vegetables delivered to your door each week.

The best sort of food is:

■ Fresh

■ Unadulterated

■ Local

■ Simple

■ Well cooked

If you've got a garden, grow some fruit and vegetables of your own and get your child involved. If you don't have a garden you can still grow some salad leaves and herbs on a balcony or windowsill, or better still get an allotment where the whole family can enjoy the outdoors and get some exercise.

Make meals an occasion

This is not about getting the best china out every night, but think about making one meal a week into a special occasion where you can sit down at a table together. You can make it as fancy as you like, but try to get everyone involved in helping, whether it's cooking, setting the table or clearing away.

Smart moves in the supermarket

Most people do their weekly shop in a supermarket and generally buy the same kind of things week in week out. You will need to take a long look at what goes in your trolley if you want to start helping your child.

Supermarkets have been criticised in the past for promoting unhealthy foods to children, limiting choice and encouraging over consumption of the wrong type of food. But under pressure from the government they have become very aware of the part they play and if you know what to look for, there's a lot of helpful information available. Next time you shop, ask about low fat and reduced sugar ranges. See what information they have or ask where you can get more.

Reading between the labels

Most packaged foods now sold in supermarkets will have a panel on the label showing basic nutritional information, including Guideline Daily Amounts (GDA) and an ingredients list. The Food Standards Agency has devised a 'traffic light' system that many supermarkets, although not all, have adopted. This information, whichever system the supermarket is using, means you can tell at a glance what's in the food. Check out which system the supermarket you shop in uses and try to familiarise yourself with the basics.

For more information on the 'traffic light' system, go to www.food.gov.uk.

What's a little, what's a lot?

You can also use the basic nutritional information as a quick way of working out whether the particular food is right for you.

A lot of fat is 20 grams or more per 100 grams

A little fat is 3 grams per 100 grams

A lot of sugar is 10 grams per 100 grams

A little sugar is 2 grams or less per 100 grams

Anything in between is moderate, so you know what to avoid.

Watch out for meaningless descriptions

Although the law requires food manufacturers to be honest on their packaging, some of the food descriptions can still be misleading, so watch out for phrases like:

- Fat free/low fat
- No added sugar
- Helps maintain a healthy diet
- Fresh, natural
- Extra fruit

These don't tell you anything useful about the food, for example something that is fat free could contain a lot of sugar which would make it fattening.

Leave it on the shelf

Here are some things that you should phase out from your child's diet as soon as possible – just leaving these things on the shelf will have a positive impact on your child's weight.

Fizzy drinks

The soft drinks industry is worth about £5 billion in Britain and many of the consumers are children. Although these drinks contain little more than empty calories and additives, children and teenagers in particular get attached to their favourite brand and it's difficult to separate the two.

Many of these drinks are sold in a minimum half litre bottle and contain as much energy as a small meal, so a child who drinks one with lunch will be filling up on a high calorie and high sugar cocktail and probably won't want to eat any food.

Try to cut back as much as possible by allowing your child to have a small glassful of their favourite drink, if they insist, at the end of the meal. You could also try to substitute this with a low sugar flavoured water or fizzy mineral water. Don't buy super size bottles of fizzy drinks and try to stop your child from glugging these drinks down between meals.

'Many of these drinks are sold in half litre bottles and contain as much energy as a small meal, so a child who drinks one with lunch will be filling up on a high calorie and high sugar cocktail and probably won't want to eat any food.'

Pies, pastries, cakes, biscuits and sausage rolls

A word of caution about pastries and cakes, as these foods tend to be very high in fat and sugar and there's no way of telling what's in them. Children love the flaky pastry of sausage rolls, pies and pastries but you will need to avoid giving these out as snacks between meals. Save the cakes and biscuits for after a meal and serve the savouries as part of a main meal.

Facts about fats

You may have heard about 'good' and 'bad' fats. So, what's the difference?

Saturated fat is the type that can increase the risk of heart disease because it raises cholesterol. This fat is found in pies, sausages, cakes and biscuits, and should be avoided.

One of the real nasties is trans fat, which has been in the news a lot lately. This is a form of vegetable oil which has been processed to turn it into a long life fat. It is used to bulk out sweets, biscuits, ready meals and cakes. Trans fat has no nutritional value and sometimes appears on labelling as 'hydrogenated oil'.

Look out for this and avoid it. Evidence about the health problems it causes - from heart disease and stroke to fertility problems - is stacking up. Trans fats are banned from food use in some countries but not the UK, although some supermarkets are phasing them out.

Sweets and treats

Children's pocket money seems to go a long way and for a few pence they can buy bumper bags of sweets and bargain bars of chocolate. It's not realistic to expect your child to give up their weekly sweets but try to limit them to small amounts after meals. Discourage friends and relatives from buying them for your child and make sure you don't use them as treats or rewards, so your child doesn't associate them with good behaviour. If you keep them out of the house, you'll avoid temptation!

Crisps

The British Heart Foundation launched a campaign recently to demonstrate the fact that children who eat a packet of crisps a day will be consuming about a litre of oil a year. Crisps also have a high salt content, additives and even sugar. Don't make these a daily staple - try not to let children snack on them, offer an alternative for lunch boxes, split a packet between two or three or serve on the side of a meal with a salad.

Summing Up

- Take up cooking.
- Small steps make for big progress.
- Get smart in the supermarket.
- Cut back on fizzy drinks and crisps.
- Start reading the labels.

Chapter Seven

Making Healthy Eating Happen

Planning and preparing healthy meals and snacks

Good intentions aren't always enough to keep your child on course. Although you all may be very keen to start with, you will need to plan your food so that your new habits become routine and a normal part of daily family life.

Let's look at some of the practicalities of de-junking your life and getting into better eating. If you generally rush around the supermarket on auto-pilot, grabbing the same old favourites and stocking up with handy snacks and special offers, whether you want them or not, you might want to spend a bit of time planning for what you buy.

Shopping for success

Before setting foot in the supermarket, plan your meals for the week ahead; work out your main courses, side dishes, desserts, snacks and lunch box food. Use the 'meal planner' overleaf to help you.

Be fairly detailed and think about your child's food diary and anything they might have suggested changing to you. Don't be too ambitious at first but make a shopping list and try to stick to it.

Meal Planner

	Mon	Tues	Wed	Thurs	Fri	Sat	Sun
Breakfast							
Midday (inc lunch box food)							
Evening							
Snacks							

Do get a few healthy alternative snacks such as crackers, breadsticks, low fat spreads, raisins and other dried fruit and nuts (assuming no nut allergy) that you can start to offer as alternatives to chocolate, biscuits, sweets and crisps.

Use your child's FAP to help substitute and eventually run down the supplies of unhealthy foods in your house.

If you make a gradual change to healthy foods, it should be easier for your child to adapt, particularly if your child is offering the suggestions. Don't worry about your child's reactions too much at this stage, keep cool and don't make a fuss, just offer the alternatives as often as it takes. Keep substituting the unhealthy stuff with things your child has agreed to try.

Some ideas to get you started

There's no shortage of recipes and food suggestions around and you might like to try the British Nutrition Foundation, which has some great recipes available on line and by post.

Here are some child friendly, quick recipes and ideas to get you going.

Breakfast

Breakfast is not negotiable for children who want to eat healthily. Here are some ideas you might like to try:

- Reduced sugar cereal (using semi-skimmed milk for over twos) – try to include a small serving of chopped fruit, eg, apples, bananas or strawberries, either on the cereal or as a side dish.

- Try introducing a glass of unsweetened juice.

- Poached egg on wholemeal toast - add some chopped cucumber sticks or sliced tomatoes.

- Porridge – you can microwave to save time but use semi-skimmed milk and honey or low sugar jam to serve. Add some fruit on top or on the side.

- Smoothie – this won't take long to make in a blender. Use bananas, strawberries or whatever soft fruit you have to hand, and make with semi-skimmed milk.

'Don't worry about your child's reaction too much at this stage, keep cool and don't make a fuss, just offer the alternatives as often as it takes. Keep substituting the unhealthy stuff with things your child has agreed to try.'

Quick lunch

Here are some suggestions for weekends or school holidays when you need something quick and tasty:

- Cheese toastie – use a low fat cheese and add a few salad leaves or a couple of olives on the side, or a couple of spoonfuls of coleslaw.

- Lentil soup with wholemeal bread.

- Home-made hummus & pitta bread strips with sliced cucumber, carrot and pepper sticks.

Evening or more substantial midday meal

Here are some evening or main meal ideas. Serve with salad or steamed vegetables:

- Baked potato - microwave for speed and fill with low fat cheese, coleslaw or baked beans.

- Home-made chicken nuggets - use the recipe provided, ditch the chips and serve with rice.

- Easy to make pizza - use the recipe provided, and your child can put their own pizza together. Let them create their own toppings.

- Macaroni cheese or cauliflower cheese - you can use a sauce mix for the cheese but check the ingredients to ensure there are no hidden nasties.

Side dishes

Try to include two or three accompaniments to each main dish as they will give your child a varied diet and balance the meal:

- Cous cous, rice and bulgur wheat are really good in place of chips.

- Dry roasted slices of potatoes or boiled new potatoes.

- Leaf salad - children may find a bunch of salad leaves or rocket easier to handle than a full blown salad. You can introduce cherry tomatoes and dress with lemon.

- Steamed vegetables - choose whatever vegetables your child will eat and steam lightly so they are crisp and crunchy.

- Corn on the cob, or heated tinned corn if you're in a hurry.

Afters

Here are some healthier puddings you could offer:

- Fruit - let children choose from a bowl of fresh fruit or share a bunch of juicy grapes between the family.

- Fruit salad - make your own from apples, strawberries, kiwis, grapes - whatever you have to hand. Use juice to sweeten and serve with low fat ice cream.

- Low fat yoghurts or low fat chocolate dessert – but make sure they are not loaded with sugar.

Drinks

Water is best with a meal but you could also offer fresh juice or a smoothie, which would count towards their five a day. If your child won't give up fizzy drinks, allow one small glass but encourage them to try carbonated water or a fruit flavoured water.

Super quick ideas

For people who are really busy:

- Stir fry - this can be put together in minutes with diced chicken or lean beef, and supermarket stir fry mix and noodles. Use tofu as a vegetarian alternative.

- Caesar salad - use a bag of salad leaves and a hot ready roasted chicken, strip off the white meat and mix with salad. Toast a slice of wholemeal bread for croutons and use low fat dressing.

- Chef's salad - slice up cold meats and cheese and add to salad leaves for a main meal. Use low fat salad dressing to drizzle.

- Omelette - try to master making a good omelette and then add any type of vegetable or cooked meat and serve as a main course.

- Toppings on toast - fast but simple. For a quick evening meal, choose from a poached egg, beans, cheese or any healthy option. Serve on wholemeal toast with sliced tomato.

Portion sizes

One of the theories about the sharp increase in obesity is that portion sizes have got bigger all round, and we now want and expect far more on our plates than ever before. Don't overload your child's plate and consider using small side plates to make food look more. They can always ask for second helpings!

Your own ready meals

To save time, and to ensure you always have something healthy to hand, make large amounts of food, such as soups, chillies, curries and pasta sauces. These can all be frozen in handy portions.

Don't be too saucy

Using ketchup, gravy, mayo, salad dressings and sauces may make the food more attractive to your child but it will also add salt, fat, sugar and sometimes more additives than you know what to do with. Check the labels and go for low fat, reduced salt varieties and use sparingly.

My child's a fussy eater

It seems that children have never been fussier about what they eat. Most of them have a list of likes and dislikes as long as history. The fact is, children are not born with food preferences any more than they are born wanting to wear a seat belt. Just as you wouldn't let your child ride in a car without a seat belt, why allow them to eat food that can harm them?

When a child says 'I don't like cheese' they will be thinking of a time when they ate a particular piece of cheese and didn't enjoy it. It's better if parents don't encourage their children to develop faddy habits by accepting what they say. If you give your child the food they want, you risk creating a vicious circle.

It's up to you to encourage your child to keep trying new varieties of foods, and in different combinations. Everyone has likes and dislikes but unless there is a genuine food allergy then there's no reason not to experiment.

Dealing with fussy eaters isn't easy and it's frustrating to start off with, but here are some suggestions:

- Decide whether your child's fussy eating is just a bid to get your attention. Work with your child on their food diary so they feel involved in choosing food.

- Try not to think about all the things your child won't eat. Look at what they will eat and build on it - don't let them reject things without trying them first.

- Set up your own café - you may have told your children lots of times 'This is not a café' but you could run your kitchen like a café for a week. Set a weekly menu, and opening times, employ the children to prepare food, wait on tables, wash up and clear away. They'll have so much fun that they'll forget their fussy eating.

- Do blind tasting - get your child to try small pieces of fruit, vegetables or cheese and see if they can identify it. They might even get a taste for it!

- Surprise snack games - put food items in a bag and allow your child to pick a snack without seeing it. Use a variety of snacks, but ensure your child eats what they pull out.

'The fact is, children are not born with food preferences any more than they are born wanting to wear a seat belt.'

Snack attack

According to the 'Sodexho School Meals and Lifestyle Survey', children spent nearly £190 million on sweets, drinks, chocolate and confectionery in 2005. Snacks may be small but the wrong types can easily derail a healthy eating plan.

Children love crisps, sweets and chocolate but you really need to limit their intake. If you don't stock up on sweets and treats, your child won't be tempted!

Look for healthier varieties and replace crisps or chocolate, with fruit. To lessen the impact, do this a couple of times a week at first. It won't be easy as snacks are now a big part of being a child but here are some ideas that might help:

- Buy some individual plastic containers to fill with dried fruit, raisins, apricots, and nuts, if appropriate, for after school snacking.
- Switch to low fat, salt and sugar products and try to buy in smaller quantities. It's not the end of the world if you run out.
- Try crisp breads, rice cakes, oatcakes, bread sticks and crackers with low fat cheese.
- Low fat popcorn is a good idea - children will love seeing it made if you buy some unpopped.
- Smoothies are filling - use milk, bananas and other soft fruit to whizz up one of these.
- Wholemeal toast spread thinly with low fat spread is a quick and filling snack.
- Try to get out of the habit of giving children sweets and treats for rewards, to stop the association with good behaviour.

Packed lunches

Packed lunches are popular with children and schools and should be a good opportunity for parents to ensure their children are given healthy options at lunchtime.

The Food Standards Agency estimates that children in the UK eat over 5.5 billion lunch boxes every year - almost three-quarters of these contain crisps, and only half contain fruit.

It's convenient to buy pre-packed stuff to fill a lunch box, but you're missing the chance to give your child a healthy balance when they need it most.

Going back to the healthy plate, it's easy to achieve a healthy balance by being careful.

Include these:

- Fruit and vegetables – at least one proportion. This could be a salad, a carrot or fruit.
- Meat or fish - tuna is a good option but you could also use cold meat on a wholemeal roll or hummus as a vegetarian alternative.
- Starchy food - this should be included everyday in the form of bread, rice or pasta.
- Milk and dairy - don't buy processed cheese, instead use dough cutters to make your own shapes. Include skimmed milk or a low fat yoghurt.
- Drinks - this could be water or a smoothie.

Give these a miss:

- Fizzy drinks.
- Chocolate and sweets.
- Pies and pastries.
- Crisps and salted roasted nuts.

Away from home

If your child is away from home at a relative's house, at an after school club or in organised childcare, it's best to get these carers on board with what you are trying to do. If necessary, pack a healthy lunch box for your child so they don't need to eat the foods they are trying to avoid.

It won't be the end of the world if your child goes to a party where sausage rolls, chips and cakes are all that is on offer, as long as they are eating healthily at home. Give your child a healthy snack before setting off so they are not tempted too much and get into the habit of carrying fruit or healthy alternatives for when you're out and about.

You should also make sure you carry a bottle of water around, so fizzy drinks do not tempt your child.

If you are out and about looking for lunch, avoid the chip shop and the takeaways – buy bread rolls, cheese and fruit from the supermarket for a picnic.

Quick and easy recipes

Smoothies

To make one large smoothie use half a pint of semi-skimmed milk, one banana, three or four strawberries and any other soft fruit you fancy. Blend for 30 seconds. Do not sweeten. Serves one.

Low fat coleslaw

1 medium onion

1 large carrot

Quarter of white or red cabbage

Lemon juice

Low fat mayonnaise

Finely chop the onion and red cabbage, and put into a bowl. Grate the carrot, add two tablespoons of mayo, a tablespoon of lemon juice and season to taste. Use on sandwiches, as a side dish, with salads or with a baked potato. Serves five.

Lentil soup

1 medium onion

1 mug of red lentils

1 low salt chicken or vegetable stock cube

2 tablespoons of tomato puree

1 tablespoon of sunflower oil

Wash and drain lentils. Finely chop the onion and fry in oil until soft. Add the lentils and seasoning to the pan and add a pint of stock. Dissolve the puree in mug of hot water and add to the pan. Bring to the boil and simmer vigorously for 30 minutes until lentils have dissolved. Blend if you want a smoother soup. Serves five.

Easy hummus

1 can of chickpeas (drained)

1 tablespoon of tahini paste

Juice of 1 lemon

1 tablespoon of olive oil

Put all the ingredients into a bowl and blend. If the mixture seems too dry, add some of the water drained from the can until you get a creamy paste. Serve with pitta bread and carrot and pepper sticks. Serves five.

Easy Pizza

Dough

8oz self raising flour

6 tablespoons of milk

1 tablespoon of oil

Tomato sauce

Passata or creamed tomatoes

Garlic

Salt & pepper

Low fat mozzarella

> 'If you make these properly, children will never want to eat the frozen ones again!'

Mix the flour, milk and oil in a bowl, turn out onto a wooden board and knead. Cover and leave to rest for 10 minutes. Roll the dough out into two seven-inch cake tins or a 10-inch pizza plate. Cover with tomato sauce, passata, garlic, seasoning and mozzarella. Cook in medium oven for 15-20 minutes. Serves five.

Home-made chicken nuggets

2 or 3 skinless chicken breasts

3 or 4 tablespoons of plain flour - seasoned with salt and pepper

2 slices of dried wholemeal bread - blended into fine breadcrumbs

1 egg - blended

Oil for frying

Cut the chicken into cubes or strips. Roll the chicken in the flour then dip in the egg. Put the chicken straight into the breadcrumbs and make sure all surfaces are well coated. Fry in shallow low fat oil until golden and drain on kitchen paper. Serve with side salad, coleslaw, rice or dry roast potatoes. Serves five.

Fruit salad

Chop apples, grapes, kiwis, strawberries and any other fruit you have to hand into a bowl. Use a dash of lemon juice to keep the fruit fresh and a glass of orange juice to sweeten. Serve with ice cream. Serves five.

Stick with it

Although it may seem like an uphill struggle, don't give up - even if your first efforts only result in cutting back a packet of crisps and a fizzy drink a week, it's worth it and you can build on it. The habits of a lifetime are hard to break, but make sure your child knows why you are doing this and that you will keep trying.

Summing Up

- Plan your meals and snacks for the week ahead.

- Master a few simple and easy recipes.

- Fussy eaters are created not born.

- Don't give up, a minor change is better than nothing.

Chapter Eight

Getting Active, Staying Active

Keeping active is important for everyone, regardless of age, shape or size, but for children and young people it is the key to their current and future health. Experts agree that healthy eating alone is not enough to control weight or build up fitness – your child needs to be active!

Being active will help your child to:

- Grow well and develop strong bones.

- Have healthy heart and lung functions.

- Control medical conditions, such as asthma.

- Reach a good 'energy balance' by burning excess calories and increasing metabolic rate.

- Avoid risk of heart disease by reducing high blood pressure and cholesterol.

- Achieve good self-esteem through setting goals and beating personal bests.

- Establish good activity habits, which are likely to last into adulthood and get passed on to the next generation.

- De-stress, get rid of pent up energy and sleep well.

The list just goes on! Surveys from the British Heart Foundation report, 'Couch Kids - The Continuing Epidemic', show evidence that children who are more physically active are likely to study better and be more successful at school, and active children are less likely to smoke or use illegal drugs than children who are inactive. With so many good reasons to keep active, we need to understand what's stopping children from taking part in activity.

Active or inactive?

Everyone assumes that the children of today are much less active than in previous generations, but this isn't the full story. A survey by the British Heart Foundation into children's lifestyles, found a fairly positive picture of exercise and activity among children and young people in the UK, with high percentages of children hitting the 60 minutes a day target.

These positive figures, however, just aren't enough to be effective against the fizzy drinks and energy overloaded snacks that children now consume. This is further evidence that the only effective way to tackle obesity is by cutting out certain types of foods and increasing activity. Although 60 minutes is the recommended daily requirement, it is only a minimum and may not be enough for some children.

Some children are more at risk than others

The British Heart Foundation study also identified certain groups of children that were less likely to achieve the desired amount of daily activity than others. Adolescent girls are one group who were not reaching 60 minutes a day, as were children from less well off backgrounds.

Children from ethnic minority backgrounds, particularly Afro Caribbean and South Asian, were also less active than their counterparts in the white community, despite being more likely to be overweight or obese.

Child's eye view

It's tempting to think that children's inactivity can be put down to too much TV but research suggests children are much more switched on to healthy activity than most people would imagine. Children are more positive about exercise

'The 2002 Health Survey for England found that, among 2-15 year-olds, 70% of boys and 61% of girls took part in 60 minutes of physical activity, seven days a week outside of school hours. The 1998 Scottish Health Survey showed similar findings for both boys and girls.'

and keeping fit than they are about healthy eating, and they value sport and activity as a means of having a good time, meeting friends and keeping healthy.

So what's standing in their way?

If children are as keen on fitness and activity as they say, it should in theory be easy to get them fired up and ready to go. However, it's not always that straightforward. What's holding them back?

- Parents not leading active lives and not helping to get their children involved.

- Lack of safe places to play locally - children and parents may feel strangers, older children and traffic pose too much of a risk.

- Lack of suitable activities - if all that's available are selective, competitive team games, non-sporty types will switch off.

- Lack of time or other options - children have lots of exciting options to choose from now or simply don't have time.

- Parents not allowing their children to get involved in activities because of their own time constraints and busy family lives.

What should I do?

As a parent, you need to understand that you have an important role to play in encouraging and supporting your child's involvement in activity, and should set a good example by keeping active yourself. Encourage your child not to spend so much time in front of the television or the computer, and get involved together in regular weekend activities.

Pull the plug on too much TV

It's estimated that 28 per cent of children in the UK watch more than four hours of TV a day - and why wouldn't they, with wall to wall children's channels and such a wide choice? In this case, for children trying to control their weight, it's not what you do, but what you don't do, that's important.

If many parents are honest, they will admit that they value TV time as it keeps the children quiet and allows them to get their own things done. Although children need down time, you should try to negotiate a reduction in viewing hours. Try swapping half an hour of TV for an activity to add towards their 60 minutes a day.

How can we build up to 60 minutes a day?

Government guidelines say that children should do at least 60 minutes of 'moderate intensity' activity a day. This could be brisk walking, cycling or playground games. It doesn't have to be done in one go and the activities your child can do to build up to the full 60 minutes can be varied - playing in the park, walking, scooting, bouncing on a trampoline, dancing or skipping – the list is endless. However, this is a minimum, and as already mentioned, you might need to aim for more.

An easy way to make sure your child gets regular exercise everyday

There is an easy way to help your child reach their 60 minutes a day and that's to leave the car at home. Walking to school and back has many benefits:

- An average journey to and from school makes up for about 8-14 minutes of activity everyday.
- Boys who walk to school are more active after school and in the evening, compared to those who travel by car.
- Children aged 12-13 use more calories in a week walking to and from school than they do in two hours of PE.
- Children who walk to school are more likely to play sport.

It's interesting that obesity rates have been rising as long as walking to school has been decreasing. However, everyone wins if you leave the car at home, and less congestion around the school makes the journey to school safer.

If there are compelling reasons for you to drive, see if there is a 'walking bus' for your child to join or park away from the school and let your child walk the last few minutes.

Stick to your FAP

By now you shouldn't need any more convincing of the benefits of keeping active, but to start your child off, it's useful to go back to the Food and Activity Plan to see how your child can work out what to do and when. Just fill in the diary and choose some aims on a weekly basis and work out if they have been achieved at the end of the week. Do this for as long as you feel you need to.

Choosing the right kind of activity for your child

Just as you need to be tactful when talking to your child about weight and obesity, you need to be very sensitive to what your child feels comfortable with as regards exercise and activity. Swimming is great but if your child is self-conscious about their body then avoid it. Even if you just go for a brisk walk around the park to start with, it's something to build on. The key thing is to start with small gradual steps that your child can build on and progress with. Here are some ideas:

- Skateboarding
- Scooting
- Cycling
- Walking
- Climbing
- Swimming
- Trampoline
- Football kick about
- Walking the dog
- Frisbee
- Hula-hoop
- Ice skating
- Rollerblading

- Badminton
- Tennis
- Hike
- Skipping
- Games in the garden

You won't be able to do outdoor activities throughout the year, so make sure there are indoor ones you can do in winter. See if your child would like to join a class, for example, judo or martial arts, so they can do an activity on a regular basis.

Tips for engaging your child and building up to 60 minutes a day

- Invest in a pedometer so your child can time or count steps, do time trials and beat personal bests. You can also use the calorie counter to show how much energy your child is burning.

- Aim to make smooth progress, letting your child control the pace. Try to introduce challenging new activities and keep pushing the boundaries to get a sense of achievement.

- Don't forget to have fun! You're not training for the Olympic Games so make sure that whatever you are doing, whether it's a walk in the rain, a game of cricket, or hula hooping in the back garden, it's as relaxed and enjoyable as possible.

- Try to build physical activity into your everyday family life. Walk when you can, play games in the garden or visit the park on your way home from school.

- If you can find another child to join in, so much the better. This will help increase your child's motivation and enthusiasm.

- If you're comfortable with your child being out in the neighbourhood, send them round the block on a scooter or bike.

'Just as you need to be tactful when talking to your child about weight and obesity, you need to be very sensitive to what your child feels comfortable with as regards exercise and activity.'

■ Don't forget to reward and recognise your child's achievements, give them small presents such as sports equipment or clothing, and aim to build up to other more exciting activities.

What can other organisations do to help?

It's worth finding out what all the organisations your child comes into contact with can do for you. Speak to your child's school to see if there are any more activities they could get involved in. Ask if your primary school encourages activity at break and lunchtimes and whether your secondary school has any good lunchtime clubs running.

Organisations like Sport England, Sport Scotland, Sport Northern Ireland and the Sports Council for Wales are worth investigating as they should have advice and information on any special activities for children in your area.

If your child is in day care or has a child minder, or is visiting a relative, ask them if they would help you by keeping your child active. You should also see what's available for children in your local leisure or community centre.

Summing Up

- Being active will benefit your child's health now and in the future.
- Remove barriers that may be stopping your child from getting active.
- Get out of the car and away from the screen.
- Use your FAP.
- Be sensitive to your child's feelings about activity, exercise and sport.

Chapter Nine

What Does Success Look Like?

What will children get out of this?

So far we've looked at all the bad things that can happen to overweight and obese children, but here are some of the good things to look forward to. By adopting a healthy diet and getting active your child will be able to:

- Play sports and run about better.

- Concentrate more at school.

- Have healthier teeth, skin and hair.

- Not get out of breath or puff and pant.

- Gain better control of conditions such as asthma.

- Play more energetic games with friends.

- Fit into clothes for their age.

- Be protected from bad diseases in adulthood.

- Learn about good food and nutrition.

- Be more confident and comfortable with their body shape.

It's important that children understand what they are aiming for and that they are not just embarking on a weight control stint, but establishing healthy eating and activity patterns that will last a lifetime.

A confidence booster for low self esteem

Many parents report that one of the spin-offs that their children gain from embarking on weight control and activity, is increased self-confidence.

Although we've looked at lack of exercise and the 'obesigenic environment' as the main causes of obesity, many children will overeat for other reasons. A child lacking in confidence, or whose family are experiencing problems, may turn to food for comfort. Feelings of inadequacy, loneliness and anxiety can all lead to comfort eating and unwanted weight gain. This becomes a self-defeating vicious circle, as overeating and weight gain will cause a further loss of self-esteem and isolation.

For many children, the experience of tackling their condition and seeing that they can make positive changes to their own lives gives them a feeling of strength and confidence. Some children may benefit from getting involved in a formal group, as meeting others in the same boat and seeing how they tackle obesity can act as an incentive.

Getting special help

If you've tried to lose weight without any special support and have failed, or you are just not confident in being able to give your child the expert support and advice needed, then you might want to think about getting in touch with some specialists who can help you.

This doesn't mean that someone else is going to take over the responsibility for your child - you will still need to be as involved and supportive as before, but there are many advantages to using expert support:

- Your child may respond better to someone from outside the family.

- The advice you get will be up-to-date and appropriate.

- Both you and your child will have a source of support.

- Your child is likely to be more committed to their goals.

Finding out what's available

The scale of the obesity problem in the UK means that there's no shortage of health carers working in this area, and there are many options for children, ranging from obesity clinics to special residential holidays and camps. However, there's no national or regional standard for treating obesity in the UK and every area has its own schemes and projects.

The sort of help that is available will depend very much on where you live, although projects do seem to be more concentrated in major cities. What's available in your area and how you go about enrolling your child at a clinic or club depends on what sort of services are provided and paid for in your health board area.

Talk to your health care team about the available options, and discuss them with your child.

How long will we need to do this for?

The simple answer to this is that it takes as long as it takes. You will be setting off on a healthy eating and activity programme that lasts a lifetime, so there won't be any stage at which you'll stop and return to old habits.

If your child is traumatised by the possibility of all their favourite snacks and treats being snatched away, explain that you're not banning anything, just cutting back and substituting. Explain that they can still have these things, but there are going to be some new approaches to food and activity.

Use the FAD and the FAP for as long as they are useful to your child, but don't labour them if the novelty is wearing off. It could be useful to keep using some aspects of them or to revisit them if your child slips back.

The novelty of the process may keep your child interested for the first two or three weeks, but you will need to keep the motivation going for as long as it takes the good eating and activity habits to take hold and become a normal part of everyday life.

Make sure your own expectations are realistic - value every step your child takes towards becoming healthier. A child will find it very de-motivating if they think you are disappointed.

'What's available in your area and how you go about enrolling your child at a clinic or club depends on what sort of services are provided and paid for in your health board area.'

No going back

Make sure your child realises that there is no going back. In the same way as giving up smoking or becoming a vegetarian, adopting a healthy lifestyle is not something that can be reversed. There are no half measures and your child can't be 'a bit healthy', but will need to be entirely committed. Try to get your child to think of themselves as a pioneer or trendsetter and see if you can get family and friends to follow suit.

Managing your child's expectations and dealing with other people's

It is understandable that your child may be expecting to see dramatic results quite swiftly, and their friends might also be expecting some sort of radical transformation. People will be sizing your child up and looking for changes.

Children are not known for their patience but it might be off putting if you are taking things slowly and there is pressure from friends and family to see results. A solution to this could be to make sure that your child does change week on week, by getting a new haircut or new items of clothing. At least there will be visible changes which will take attention away from losing weight.

Giving up and slipping up

You should prepare yourself for your child giving up and slipping up along the way. It would be very unusual for a child to drop all their old inactive habits and not get cravings for certain foods. As long as you have established what you are doing and why you are doing it, and they are in basic agreement, then a few detours from the main path shouldn't make such a big difference.

How to keep your child positive and motivated:

- Remain positive and upbeat.
- Keep reminding them of why they are doing this and where they want to be.

- Keep on with the healthy eating but try to vary it a bit if the menu is getting boring.

- Keep on with the activities but try to introduce some variety.

- Remind them of things they did really well and can do again.

You might want to arrange a special activity, family outing or even visit someone who has done a similar thing successfully. This is where the support of the whole family is so important - if you are all backing your child and can come up with ways of keeping them on track, they are likely to carry on.

It's helpful if you can be positive about what you're doing so your child doesn't see this as an exercise in being deprived of their favourite things. Point out how much better they look or how much more energy they have.

Shock tactics

Although it's never a good idea to shock or frighten children into losing weight, if you think your child is interested and they would benefit from it, talk to them about the food they are craving. Use facts; explain how it's made and the risks. Don't labour the point or demonise certain types of foods, but once children know the facts about something, they may respond differently to it.

Rewarding positive behaviour

Keep the fact that you are not doing this to ban your child from eating their favourite foods at the front of the conversation. It's important your child understands that what you are doing is in their interests. Make sure your child understands this by:

- Praising them when they do something right.

- Keeping the positive encouragement going.

- Reminding them of a time they did something really well.

- Showing them you have confidence in them.

'It's helpful if you can be positive about what you're doing so your child doesn't see this as an exercise in being deprived of their favourite things.'

Younger children especially may benefit from using a star chart system so they can track their progress. But for both older and younger children, you can use the points from the FAP to reward them.

You could let older children trade points for rewards, so that if they reach a total of 10 points in a particular week, they can exchange this for a trip to the cinema or something similar. It's up to you how you want to work it but if children can see the rewards in concrete terms, they are likely to be more motivated. Once they've achieved one 'prize', they're likely to keep going for another.

It's up to you to help your child

Ultimately parents are the best people to help their child beat the obesity time bomb. You will have helped teach your child to do many things in life such as getting dressed, crossing the road, learning to read or riding a bike. This is no different, but it's a lot more serious. Your child will be depending on you to make sure that they aren't among the 25 per cent of children who will be obese by the year 2050.

Summing Up

■ Make sure your child stays motivated and on track.

■ Be prepared for slipping back to bad habits.

■ Keep rewarding and recognising your child's achievements.

■ Parents are the best people to help their child beat obesity.

Help List

Where to go for further information

Before starting to make changes to your child's lifestyle your first port of call should be your local health centre or doctor's surgery, where you will be able to find the latest information and contacts. What help is available will vary according to where you live.

It's important to speak to someone in your local health care team, either your GP, a health visitor or practice nurse, as they know more about your child's health than anyone. This is particularly important if your child has any other medical conditions. Your health care team will be able to advise you and recommend the options open to your child.

You could also ask your local pharmacist for advice and information, or contact your child's school and see if the school nurse can offer any advice and support.

For fitness activities, try your local leisure centre. Find out if they provide any special facilities for children trying to control their weight. They could have special schemes, courses or reduced prices for young people.

Community centres often organise special activities or are used by people running their own clubs for children. If you can't see anything suitable why not try and start a class of your own? Get together with other parents to organise an activity - it could be basketball, judo, cheerleading, aerobics or anything your child would like.

The web is a good source of information but you will need to be selective and work out which sites are more useful than others. Some sites have areas specially designed to appeal to children and young people. If you find something you think would help your child, let them see it but don't insist if they are not interested.

There are too many organisations concerned with health and child obesity to list but the following will be a good starting point.

General information

Association for the Study of Obesity (ASO)

20 Brook Meadow Close, Woodford Green, Essex, IG8 9NR
Tel: 020 8503 2042
www.aso.org.uk
The Association for the Study of Obesity (ASO) was founded in 1967 and is dedicated to the understanding and treatment of obesity. It aims to promote awareness of obesity and its impact on health, research and understanding of the causes, prevention and treatment of obesity. Although the site is not aimed at parents, there is good advice, useful links and contacts.

BBC Science and Nature, Hot Topics Child Obesity

www.bbc.co.uk
Worth a look around the BBC website and at the Science and Nature section in particular. There is a lot of general, factual, newsy information for parents, and some sections are aimed at children. It's clear, concise and tells you and your child everything you need to know.

Carnegie Weight Management

Tel: 0113 283 2600 ext 25233
www.carnegieweightmanagement.com
Carnegie Weight Management provides education, training and research to treat overweight and obese children. The programme involves a range of treatments which have been developed and tested to target and successfully treat child obesity. The organisation runs weight loss camps and organises clubs for children.

The Children's Weight Clinic

PO Box 28533, Edinburgh, EH4 2WW
Tel: 07707 878789
enquiries@childrensweightclinic.com
www.childrensweightclinic.com

An independent family based clinic that promotes healthy family lifestyles and specialises in child obesity. Advises and supports families in establishing a healthier, happier lifestyle. Run by dietician Laura Stewart.

Department of Health – Obesity

Tel: 020 7210 4850
www.dh.gov.uk
The Department of Health website provides detailed information on child obesity, health and fitness. Many of the publications are downloadable or you can contact the Department of Health directly for hard copies of guides and leaflets.

Harlow Printing Limited

Maxwell Street, South Shields, Tyne & Wear, NE33 4PU
Tel: 0191 455 4286
sales@harlowprinting.co.uk
www.harlowprinting.co.uk
You can purchase the whole range of UK growth reference charts from here.

The MEND Programme

Unit 21, Tower Workshops, 58 Riley Road, London, SE1 3DG
Tel: 0870 609 1405
www.mendprogramme.org
Currently in operation in regions of England, the MEND Programme is a free after school course which helps families learn how to be fitter and healthier. MEND Programmes are open to children (aged 7 to 13) who are above their ideal weight. They must be accompanied by a parent or carer. Contact MEND for locations or news of courses starting up.

National Obesity Forum

First Floor, 6a Gordon Road, Nottingham, NG2 5LN
Tel: 0115 846 2109
info@nof.uk.com
www.nationalobesityforum.org.uk

This was established by health professionals in May 2000 to raise awareness of the growing impact that obesity was having. One of the most high profile organisations involved in obesity campaigning. A very comprehensive site and a good source of up-to-date information on nutrition and exercise for children, and where to get help.

NHS sites for different areas of the UK

Below are the relevant NHS sites for Wales, Northern Ireland, England and Scotland. These are useful gateway sites to access in depth information and support relevant to the area where you live. They all contain sections on healthy living, children's health and medical facts about the causes of obesity and the treatments available.

Northern Ireland: www.n-i.nhs.uk
Scotland: www.show.scot.nhs.uk
Wales: www.wales.nhs.uk
England: www.nhs.uk

Patient UK

www.patient.co.uk

A UK medical information website for patients. It provides good quality information about health and disease on a wide range of medical and health topics. It also reviews health related websites and links to many of these from the web directory included. Also lists support groups, charities and therapists.

NHS WATCH IT

Belmont House, 3-5 Belmont Grove, Leeds, LS2 9DE
Tel: 0113 392 6352

WATCH IT is an award winning, Leeds based, NHS programme designed to help and support 8-16-year olds who have difficulty with their weight. It is now being offered nationally as a training programme and will be of particular interest to primary healthcare organisations, local councils and all those involved in public health.

Weight Concern

Brook House, 2-16 Torrington Place, London, WC1E 7HN
Tel: 0207 679 6636

enquiries@weightconcern.org.uk
www.weightconcern.org.uk
A UK charity committed to developing and researching new treatments for obesity and supporting self-help. No help line or individual advice offered but the website is very detailed, and includes a children's BMI calculator and lots of child specific information. It does charge for some of its publications but the website is fairly comprehensive.

Weight Loss Resources

www.weightlossresources.co.uk
Weight Loss Resources provides calorie and nutritional information. It gives you all the facts on what your body needs, and provides all the tools you need to take control, lose weight and eat well. A calorie counter and exercise diary is included.

Food

British Nutrition Foundation

High Holborn House, 52-54 High Holborn, London, WC1V 6RQ
Tel: 020 7404 6504
postbox@nutrition.org.uk
www.nutrition.org.uk
The British Nutrition Foundation provides healthy eating information, resources for schools, news items, recipes and details of the work going on around the UK. Lots of information on food and activities, and includes special sections for children.

The Food Commission

94 White Lion Street, London, N1 9PF
Tel: 020 7837 2250
enquiries@foodcomm.org.uk
www.foodcomm.org.uk

The Food Commission campaigns for the right for everyone to eat safe, wholesome, good quality food. It has also developed a website designed for independent use by secondary school students aged 11-14 or for anyone who is interested in how our food is produced and what its effect is on our health and the environment. An excellent resource for teachers is www.chewonthis.org.uk.

The Food Standards Agency

www.food.gov.uk
England: Aviation House, 125 Kingsway, London, WC2B 6NH
Tel: 020 7276 8000
Scotland: 6th Floor, St Magnus House, 25 Guild Street, Aberdeen, AB11 6NJ
Tel: 01224 285100
scotland@foodstandards.gsi.gov.uk
Northern Ireland: 10 A-C Clarendon Road, Belfast, BT1 3BG
Tel 028 9041 7700
infofsani@foodstandards.gsi.gov.uk
Wales: 11th Floor, South Gate House, Wood Street, Cardiff, CF10 1EW
Tel: 02920 678999
wales@foodstandards.gsi.gov.uk
One of the best sites and worth revisiting - if you only visit one site make it this one! Links from the homepage will take you to news and activities in Scotland, Wales and Northern Ireland. For information on food, recipes and healthy eating aimed at specific children's age groups, try FSA site www.eatwell.gov.uk.

Weight Wise Website - British Dietetic Association

www.bdaweightwise.com
This is an independent site, with unbiased, easy-to-follow hints and tips - based on the latest evidence to help you manage weight for good. It will help you take a look at your child's current eating habits and physical activity levels, and offer a practical approach to setting goals for a lifestyle change.

Parenting contacts

www.netmums.com

Netmums, 124 Mildred Avenue, Watford, WD18 7DX

contactus@netmums.com

Netmums is a local UK network for mums (and dads), offering a wealth of information on both a national and local level. You can access local support information and swap advice with other parents. Lots of good articles about healthy eating and food.

www.raisingkids.co.uk

117 Rosebery Road, London, N10 2LD
Tel: 0208 883 8621
customerservice@raisingkids.co.uk

Raising Kids is a site dedicated to parenting skills, with useful special features on food and nutrition, a discussion board, recipes and survival tactics. It also offers online discussion and expert opinion.

Exercise activity and sporting information

www.foodfitness.org.uk

C/O Food and Drink Federation, 6 Catherine Street, London, WC2B 5JJ
Tel: 020 7836 2460
foodfitness@fdf.org.uk

Food Fitness is a healthy lifestyle initiative from the Food and Drink Federation. It promotes healthy eating and increased moderate physical activity. Lots of sound advice about eating and drinking, and some fun activities for children on the site with two cartoon families, the Activators and the Dolittlers.

National Sports Agencies

These organisations are responsible for promoting sport and active lifestyles in their respective areas. They encourage people at all levels to get more involved in physical activity and are a good source of information if you are looking for advice about special activities and initiatives for children where you live.

Scotland: Sport Scotland, Caledonia House, South Gyle, Edinburgh, EH12 9DQ
Tel 0131 317 7200
library@sportscotland.org.uk
www.sportscotland.org.uk

England: Sport England, 3rd Floor Victoria House, Bloomsbury Square, London, WC1B 4SE
Tel: 020 7273 1551
info@sportengland.org
www.sportengland.org
Wales: Sports Council for Wales, Sophia Gardens, Cardiff, CF11 9SW
Tel: 0845 045 0904
scw@scw.org.uk
www.sports-council-wales.org.uk
Northern Ireland: Sport Northern Ireland, House of Sport, Upper Malone Road, Belfast BT9 5LA
Tel: 028 90 381222
info@sportni.net
www.sportni.net

Health and children's charity organisations

Children don't need to be suffering from any of the conditions that the health charities listed below are involved in. But these groups take an active interest in child obesity because they are aware of the scale of the problem and what it will mean for children's future health. They all have useful information for parents, carers and professionals relating to their specialist area. Some have eating and activity guides and useful links and contacts. Most have offices based in Wales, Northern Ireland and Scotland and some have offices in regions of England.

Barnardos

Tanners Lane, Barkingside, Ilford, Essex, IG6 1QG
Tel: 020 8550 8822
www.barnardos.org.uk

British Heart Foundation

14 Fitzhardinge Street, London, W1H 6DH
Tel: 020 7935 0185
www.bhf.org.uk

Cancer Research UK

P.O. Box 123, Lincoln's Inn Fields, London WC2A 3PX
Tel: (Supporter Services) 020 7121 6699
Tel: (Switchboard) 020 7242 0200
www.cancerresearch.org.uk

Diabetes UK

Macleod House, 10 Parkway, London NW1 7AA
Tel: 020 7424 1000
info@diabetes.org.uk
www.diabetes.org.uk

Resources for schools and teachers

British Heart Foundation Food 4 Thought Campaign

14 Fitzhardinge Street London W1H 6DH
Tel: 020 7935 0185
www.bhf.org.uk
In January 2008, the British Heart Foundation launched a new campaign aimed at fighting the obesity epidemic in children. Using the internet and special teacher's packs, the campaign encourages 11-13 year-olds to think about the food they eat and be more aware of junk food marketing tricks. An interactive website for secondary school pupils is available at www.bhf.org. uk/food4thought, which allows children to explore a virtual world and expose hidden marketing messages and food content. Teachers packs are available from BHF.

The Caroline Walker Trust

22 Kindersley Way, Abbots Langley, Herts, WD5 0DQ
Tel: 01923 445374
www.cwt.org.uk
The Caroline Walker Trust is targeted towards vulnerable groups who need special help with eating and nutrition. The charity produces guidelines, training materials and expert information on child nutrition needs in school and also on special needs nutrition. Useful for anyone involved in childcare.

Food Dudes

Bangor Food and Activity Research Unit, School of Psychology, Bangor University, Gwynedd, LL57 2AS
Tel: 01248 388201
fooddudes@bangor.ac.uk
www.fooddudes.co.uk
This is an excellent site for schools and teachers. The Food Dudes Healthy Eating Programme was developed by psychologists at Bangor University as a way of getting children to learn to like fruit and vegetables. The programme has been very successful and was recently adopted for use in every primary school in Northern Ireland.

Playground Fun

administrator@playgroundfun.org.uk
www.playgroundfun.org.uk

This is a useful site for teachers or carers of children. Playground Fun, developed from work at the University of Glasgow, aims to bring together traditional and modern playground and street games for children aged seven to nine, to encourage children to take part in physical activity through education. Lots of downloadable information on games and activities.

International resources

The American Heart Association

www.amhrt.org
This site contains sections for parents and children with advice on healthy eating and activity.

World Health Organisation

www.who.int/topics/obesity/en/
The WHO website has a special section on obesity around the world - a useful site for technical facts and figures. Lots of information and help from a global perspective.

Weight loss surgery information

British Obesity Surgery Patient Association

Tel: 08456 02 04 46
www.bospa.org.uk
BOSPA (British Obesity Surgery Patients Association) was launched in
December 2003 to provide support and information to UK patients interested
in finding out the facts about obesity surgery.

Weight Loss Surgery Information and Support

PO Box 796, Ipswich, 1P1 9GU
Tel: 0151 222 4737
www.wlsinfo.org.uk
Staffed by volunteers, Weight Loss Surgery Information and Support is a
source of information and support on weight loss surgery options in the UK.

Of all the useful contacts and resources a child will need, there is one source
above all that will be crucial in encouraging them to bring about changes in
lifestyle patterns. That source is the family and without their support, everything
else is just details and information. You have the potential to help your child
change their life for the better and to grow up and develop as a happier and
more confident person. The solution sounds easy, although achieving it won't
be, but it's worth sticking with as your child will come out of it with a healthy
future assured and renewed confidence and enthusiasm to tackle other
difficulties in life.

Appendix A

Find out how healthy your family's lifestyle is with this simple fun quiz

1. What is your normal family Sunday afternoon activity?

a. Sitting in front of a screen watching TV/playing games/surfing the web with snack and drink in hand.

b. We'd like to go to the pool but it's too cold so the kids are watching a film with a bag of popcorn.

c. A family bike ride after the kids have finished their morning sports classes and we've all had lunch together.

2. Which best describes mealtimes in your house?

a. Everyone for themselves, we all choose our favourite foods and settle down in front of the TV to eat.

b. We try to eat together but the children don't like home cooking so we give them a pizza or snack afterwards so they don't go hungry.

c. We sit down to three meals a day as a family, the children help to prepare, serve and clear away.

3. How often do you walk to or from school with your children?

a. Never, we have two cars and no time to walk as we're on our way to work.

b. We've done it a couple of times but it's hard to organise and almost nobody else does it.

c. We leave the car at home unless the weather is terrible or we really need to take it.

4. How many times a week do your children eat the recommended five a day?

a. They don't like fruit and vegetables and don't eat them.

b. I give them an apple in their lunch box and there's always fruit at home.

c. We make sure fresh fruit and vegetables are served with every meal and are given for snacks.

5. How often do you eat takeaway or fast foods?

a. Three or four times a week at least, the kids love their pizzas and trips to fast food restaurants.

b. We try to limit ourselves to once a week but they enjoy this type of food and sometimes it's just very convenient.

c. Very rarely, we might if we're out and about shopping together or on holiday, but we try to avoid eating fast food.

6. What's in your child's lunch box?

a. Crisps, bar of chocolate, can of fizzy drink, white bread sandwich, packet of sweets and processed cheese stick.

b. Crisps, cheese sandwich on white bread, which is all my child will eat, an apple, packet of biscuits and carton of juice.

c. Water, Greek salad, fruit salad, wholemeal pitta bread with cottage cheese and cucumber, dried fruit, grissini and a low fat, reduced sugar yoghurt.

7. How important is sport, activity and exercise to you and your family?

a. Very important, we subscribe to all the networks and have the latest computer games, which the kids love to play.

b. We love to watch football and rugby but my son never gets picked for the team and my teenage daughter doesn't like school sports.

c. We take the children swimming and try to get them to join in as many after school and weekend activities as possible.

8. Which best describes your weekly shop?

a. Rushing around the supermarket, piling the trolley high with bumper packs of snacks and treats for the kids. Bigger bottles of fizzy drink are better value and we love bogofs.

b. We try to be good and stick to our list but those special offers are very tempting and the kids slip stuff into the trolley.

c. We stick to our list, read the food information panels and look for low fat varieties. We avoid stocking up with snacks and treats.

Answers, what type of family are you?

Mostly As

At least you have honesty on your side, but as you probably realise, you will need to start making better choices surrounding your children's health than you made in our quiz. Your children are likely to be ticking time bombs and you need to start thinking about how you're going to defuse them before they explode.

Mostly Bs

Although your intentions are good and you know how many beans make five, you don't seem to know what to do with them. Instead of thinking about all the things you can't do, try to focus on making some changes that fit in with your lifestyle. You can start by making changes to your own life and setting a good example for your children.

Mostly Cs

No sign of any ticking time bomb in your house. You are ticking all the right boxes and making all the right choices for your children. You should be writing a book on healthy eating and activity, rather than reading one! Hopefully your children will be on board with your choices and will want to follow your good example.

Only a bit of fun

Of course this quiz is only a bit of fun and it should be obvious what the best choices are. Nobody makes choices that are as disastrous as family A and nobody is likely to be as perfect as family C. The fact is, most people would like to make better choices for their children but find it very difficult. Being a seriously overweight child who doesn't know how to make the right choices isn't fun. The main point to take away from the quiz is that it's up to us to help children make healthy choices.

Appendix B

Food and Activity Diary (FAD)

- Complete the FAD overleaf as honestly and accurately as you can.

- For the whole week write down everything your child eats.

- List all forms of activity, exercise or sport your child takes part in - this can be school PE, swimming, walking to school or even playing.

- Use the FAD for as long as it's useful to your child - but don't labour it if the novelty is wearing off.

- Used correctly the FAD will give you a picture of your child's normal eating and activity plans.

What did you eat?	Mon	Tues	Wed	Thurs	Fri	Sat	Sun
Breakfast							
Snacks							
Lunchtime							
Snacks							
Dinner							
Snacks							
Drinks							
What sort of activity did you do?							
How long did it take?							

Date: Weight:

Appendix C

Food and
Activity Plan (FAP)

- Using your FAD opposite, write down on the FAP overleaf what you think you can change about your child's lifestyle for a week.

- You can swap foods, drop foods or add a couple of healthier options - aim for some achievable swaps and substitutions in the first week.

- Make sure you include some activity each day - whether it's walking to school or bouncing on the trampoline.

- Be realistic and build up gradually.

- Remember, there's always next week!

FAP Week One

	Food Swap	Food Drop	Add Food	Activity
Monday				
Tuesday				
Wednesday				
Thursday				
Friday				
Saturday				
Sunday				

FAP Achievement Record

▪ Keep a daily record of your child's achievements on the following chart overleaf.

▪ You can give one point for each portion of fruit or vegetables your child eats and one point for each 15 minutes of activity.

▪ Include activities like dancing, walking and playing - everyday.

▪ Add the points up at the end of every week and encourage your child to beat their 'personal best'.

▪ Repeat the charts again for the next week and continue for as long as you feel it's useful.

▪ You may also like to include details of weight, BMI and waist circumference.

	Portion of fruit	Portion of vegetables	Activity and how long	Points
Monday				
Tuesday				
Wednesday				
Thursday				
Friday				
Saturday				
Sunday				

Total points for week:

Waist circumference:

End of week measurements:

Weight:

BMI:

Any changes:

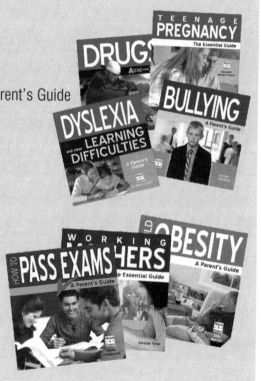